THIRD EDITION

ETHICAL DILEMMAS

IN ALLIED HEALTH

JANINE M. IDZIAK, PH.D.

LIFE SUPPORT
SHOULD WE UNPLUG?

BOY   GIRL

Kendall Hunt
publishing company

Cover image © Shutterstock.com

Kendall Hunt
publishing company

Copyright © 2000 by Simon & Kolz Publishing, LLC.

Copyright © 2010, 2016 by Kendall Hunt Publishing

PAK ISBN: 978-1-4652-9900-0
Text Alone ISBN: 978-1-5249-0272-8

Printed in the United States of America

For Carol Reffner

Contents

Preface

Over the past several decades, health care ethics has developed and flourished as an academic discipline. The field now includes a standard set of topics. Issues such as abortion, assisted reproduction, terminating life-sustaining treatment, euthanasia and physician aid-in-dying, confidentiality, and the allocation of scarce medical resources are commonly covered in textbooks on health care ethics. However, the perspective assumed in these textbooks may be limited in comparison with the actual range of health care services and types of health care professionals. Case studies on ethical dilemmas typically focus on physicians and nurses in a hospital setting.

This textbook, on the other hand, approaches the standard problems of health care ethics *from the perspective of the allied health fields.* Case studies always involve allied health professionals, giving recognition to them as an integral part of the care giving team.

Health care is no longer synonymous with the hospital setting, but includes assisted living complexes, long-term care facilities, home health care services, and hospice facilities. This book is broader in scope than many textbooks in health care ethics in including examples beyond the acute care setting.

Many health care facilities have established ethics committees to help patients, family members, and health care providers work through difficult ethical dilemmas. This textbook recognizes the increasing role ethics committees are playing in health care. It refers to the use of ethics committees and includes exercises that invite students to assume the role of ethics committee members.

Apart from the first and second background chapters, each chapter in the book has the same structure. The introductory section lists the issues to be considered in the chapter. The chapter includes one or more case studies describing concrete situations in which these issues arise, with expository sections discussing the issues. At the end of the chapter is a summary section listing key terms and concepts used in the chapter and the key points made about the issues discussed. Finally, there is a section entitled "For Further Discussion," which asks students to think critically about the material in the chapter and to apply principles they have learned to concrete cases. They are also asked to role play discussion of ethical dilemmas and to relate issues to their personal experiences. In sum, the section "For Further Discussion" invites students to become active participants in "doing ethics."

Although the case studies presented are hypothetical, they are based on particular cases or types of cases that actually occur. The case studies are generally written as if they are currently taking place. This has been done deliberately to simulate the actual ethical decision making process. When we have to make a tough ethical decision, we often do not know exactly what the outcome will be. This is part of the challenge of "doing ethics."

This textbook may be used at either the undergraduate or graduate level. Supplementary ethical, religious, and legal materials have been noted on a website and may be selected to enrich the basic printed text. The text may be used in its entirety in a course devoted specifically to ethics, or selected chapters may be used in conjunction with other courses in allied health. If the text is individualized by an instructor in this way, the selection should always include the first chapter on ethical theory and the second chapter on ethics committees.

Supplementary Resources

Kendall Hunt is providing a website to accompany this text with an Instructor's Manual and with Resources for Students. Both include additional content resources. The Instructor's Manual includes pedagogical tools as well.

Acknowledgments

As a professor of philosophy, my academic work in the field of bioethics has been greatly enriched by the "hands on" experience afforded me by serving on ethics committees at various health care facilities. In particular, I want to extend my thanks to Mercy Medical Center and Stonehill Franciscan Services in Dubuque, Iowa.

My work as a chair of the Medical-Moral Commission of the Archdiocese of Dubuque in preparing a handbook on health care ethics provided the occasion for extensive searches of the literature on bioethics. I have drawn on some of this work in preparing this textbook.

Finally, I am grateful to Loras College for granting me released time from teaching to pursue work in the field of bioethics.

Janine Marie Idziak, Ph.D.
Dubuque, Iowa
May 2016

Chapter 1

Ethics for Health Care

Ethics asks us to stand back and evaluate our actions. It asks us to judge that some actions ought to be done and that others ought to be avoided.

In the minds of some, ethics consists in nothing but a set of rules governing behavior—rules that have often been superimposed by other people. Ethics is thought of as nothing more than a list of "do's" and "don'ts."

However, contemporary philosophers have presented ethics as an enterprise fostering human happiness and fulfillment. On this view, *the purpose of ethical reflection is to consider the choices and courses of action that most promote the fulfillment of persons and the community* (1). Understood in this way, "doing ethics" is a very positive activity.

In this chapter, you will learn about:

- the distinction between clinical and organizational ethics;
- major ethical theories; and
- ethical objectivism versus ethical relativism.

1

This chapter is different from the other chapters in that it is a *reference* to which you will come back again and again as you work through the various topics in this book.

The Ethical Dimensions of Health Care

Decision making in health care often involves more than just the brute medical facts of the case. Ethical principles and values will be the determining factor in which course of action is chosen.

For example, consider decisions arising from the use of fertility drugs. Fertility drugs can result in multifetal pregnancies; that is, pregnancies where more than one fetus is conceived and carried. A famous case is that of septuplets born to the McCaugheys in Carlisle, Iowa (2). It is a medical fact that multifetal pregnancies, "particularly those which involve more than triplets, can cause health risks for the mother, such as an increased risk for hypertension, gestational diabetes, anemia, as well as the side effects from tocolytic agents often used to stop premature contractions" (2). Another medical fact is that multifetal pregnancies are risky for the babies themselves. Multifetal pregnancies frequently end in miscarriage or stillbirth, and the risk increases with the number of fetuses (3). Moreover, even when they do survive, such babies are nearly always born prematurely, with all the complications prematurity entails. Thus "multiple babies have 12 times as great a chance of dying in infancy," (3) and if they survive, they face a number of potential problems later in life, ranging from cerebral palsy to kidney and bowel problems to blindness to mental challenges (3).

Especially because of the risks to the babies themselves involved in a multifetal pregnancy, the option of "selective reduction" may be recommended. In selective reduction, several fetuses are aborted so that the remaining fetuses stand a better chance of being born healthy (3). Whether this option is chosen will depend on the couple's views about the moral permissibility of abortion. Everyone involved could agree on the medical facts of the case—the risks involved in a multifetal pregnancy. However, one couple may choose selective reduction while another couple (like the McCaugheys) may reject it because of their different views on the ethical permissibility of abortion. Their respective *ethical* views ultimately determine which course of action is taken *medically*.

Many health care facilities now have ethics committees in place (see Chapter 2). Many large health care systems employ professional ethicists to address ethical issues on a full-time basis. Just as it is a common practice to consult with specialists about medical care, so ethics consultation services are now being offered to help patients, families, and health care providers work through difficult ethical dilemmas (see Chapter 2). Thus, ethics has very much become a part of contemporary health care services.

Health care professionals should study ethics so that they can be sensitive to the ethical principles and values that enter into the decision-making processes of patients and their families. The study of ethics will likewise help prepare them to meet ethics standards set for health care facilities and by their own professional associations. Finally, studying ethics will enable health care professionals to participate fully in the ethics services offered by the facilities and agencies that employ them.

Two Levels of Ethical Inquiry in Health Care

Ethical issues concerning health care can arise at different levels. Obviously, ethical questions can arise *in the care of individual patients.* Should 80-year-old John, who has Alzheimer's disease, be resuscitated if he suffers a cardiac arrest? Should he be given antibiotics if he develops pneumonia? Eleanor has been unconscious for a year, and physicians think it very unlikely that she will ever regain consciousness. Should her tube feeding be discontinued so that she can be allowed to die? Should Jackie abort a much wanted child because prenatal diagnosis shows that her fetus has a genetic disorder? These types of questions belong to the category of *clinical ethics.*

At the same time, ethical questions can arise about *how a health care facility or service is operated.* For example, ethical questions can be raised about the financing of health care. Is it right for a physician who is part of a health maintenance organization (HMO) to refrain from prescribing a particular drug for a patient because the drug is too costly? Or, how much "charity care" should the local community hospital provide to patients who do not have the resources to pay their bills? Ethical questions can also arise regarding a health care facility's treatment of its employees. Is it appropriate for a hospital to discourage unionization on the part of its employees? Was the last merit raise for employees fairly handled? Should a married health care worker with children be dismissed if she refuses to come to work during an epidemic of an infectious disease? Yet another concern today is how the ethical value of confidentiality can be preserved with the computerization of medical records. All of these questions belong to the realm of *organizational ethics.*

While this book will give primary attention to issues in clinical ethics, some issues from the realm of organizational ethics will also be addressed.

Ethical Theories

An ethical theory is a way of organizing our ethical reflection and deliberations. It directs us to the features of a situation, which are relevant in making a determination of rightness or wrongness of action.

In this section, we offer an overview of major ethical theories, which can be brought to bear on issues in health care ethics. For each theory, we describe its standard for determining rightness and wrongness of action and give an example of how the theory applies to a particular issue.

Principlism

In *Principles of Biomedical Ethics*, a book that has now become a classic of contemporary health care ethics, Tom Beauchamp and James Childress reduce all of health care ethics to four basic principles: *autonomy, nonmaleficence, beneficence,* and *justice.* (4). These principles are sometimes referred to as the "Georgetown mantra" because of the association of the philosophers who developed them with the Kennedy Institute of Ethics at Georgetown University (4, 5).

The word "autonomy" is of Greek derivation, and "originally referred to the self-rule or self-governance of independent city-states" (4). By extension, autonomy refers to self-determination by an individual of the course of his or her own life:

> Personal autonomy encompasses, at a minimum, self-rule that is free from both controlling interference by others and from certain limitations, such as inadequate understanding that prevent meaningful choice. The autonomous individual acts freely in accordance with a self-chosen plan, analogous to the way an independent government manages its territories and establishes its policies (4).

Respecting autonomy means acknowledging *a person's right to hold views, to make choices, and to take actions based on personal values and beliefs* (4). In the context of health care, respecting autonomy means involving the patient in decisions about medical treatment, and allowing the individual to make the final decision in these matters. It also means giving the patient reasonable control and choice when interacting with the health care system in general. The principle of autonomy is related to Kantian ethics (see below) in that violating a person's autonomy "is to treat that person merely as a means; that is, in accordance with others' goals without regard to that person's own goals" (4).

The principle of nonmaleficence asserts *an obligation not to inflict harm on others* (4). In a health care context, it is associated with the maxim *primum non nocere;* that is, "above all [or first] do not harm" (4). Nonmaleficence includes "not imposing *risks* of harm," and is related to the concepts of negligence and the standard of due care (4).

Beneficence has to do with contributing to the welfare of other people, so that the principle of beneficence refers to a *moral obligation to act for the benefit of others* (4). As presented by Beauchamp and Childress, acting for the benefit or welfare of others includes preventing evil or harm, removing evil or harm, and doing or promoting good (4).

On an intuitive level, justice concerns "fair, equitable, and appropriate treatment in light of what is due or owed to persons" (4). Talk of justice often refers specifically to the concept of distributive justice, which "concerns the distribution of such social benefits and burdens as medical services, welfare payments, public offices, taxes, and military service" (6). Thus, distributive justice concerns *fairness in the distribution of social benefits and burdens* (4). As such, it encompasses fairness in the distribution of available resources. Attempts have been made to articulate more specific principles governing the distribution of social benefits and burdens. These attempts include the principle of equality, the principle of need, the principle of contribution, and the principle of effort (4, 6).

The principle of equality, as the name indicates, embodies a radical egalitarianism. Everyone is to be treated the same in all respects, and all social benefits and burdens are to be distributed equally. Everyone, so to speak, is entitled to the same slice of the pie, and everyone must bear an equal part of the social load. The principle of need is an extension of the egalitarian principle (6). According to the principle of need, goods should be parceled out according to individuals' need so that those who have greater needs receive a greater share. The outcome will be one of equality; however, for given the fact that everyone's needs will be met, everyone will end up at the same level. The treatment of individuals will be equal although the proportion of goods they receive will be different (6).

The principle of contribution, on the other hand, maintains that "everyone should get back that proportion of social goods that is the result of his or her productive labor" (6). To use an everyday example, this principle holds that "if two people work to grow potatoes and the first works twice as long or twice as hard as the second, then the first should be entitled to twice as large a share of the harvest" (6).

Finally, the principle of effort asserts that "the degree of effort made by the individual should determine the proportion of goods received by the individual." (6) Again using an everyday example, this principle holds that "the file clerk who works just as hard as the president of a company should receive the same proportion of social goods as the president" while "those who are lazy and refuse to exert themselves will receive proportionally less than those who work hard." (6). This principle is attractive in seeming to capture "our sense of what is fair—that those who do their best should be similarly rewarded, while those who do less than their best should be less well rewarded" (6).

Ethicists acknowledge that a comprehensive theory of justice may include more than one (or possibly all) of these more specific principles of distributive justice (4, 6). Indeed, it has been claimed that, as a matter of fact, "most societies invoke several of these material principles in framing public policies, appealing to different principles in different spheres and contexts" (4).

According to principlism, ethical dilemmas arise when more than one of the basic principles (autonomy, nonmaleficence, beneficence, and justice) is applicable to a situation and the principles conflict in directing what course of action ought to be taken. For example, a patient who is dying may say that she wants "everything done," including care in the intensive care unit (ICU). On the other hand, her physician may believe that ICU care would be futile in prolonging her life and might take a bed away from an emergency case coming into the hospital whose recovery would be greatly helped by ICU care. This case involves a conflict between patient autonomy and justice in the allocation of health care resources. Autonomy directs that the patient should be placed in the ICU unit. Justice, on the other hand, and more specifically, the principle of need, argues against this. The patient in an emergency situation can benefit from ICU care in a way that the terminally ill patient in question cannot, and thus can claim a greater need for ICU care. In such cases of conflict, a judgment must be made as to which principle (autonomy or justice) is weightier and should take precedence in that particular situation (4). The principle that takes precedence determines the ethically right thing to do.

One challenge in using the ethical theory of principlism is making such determinations of precedence in a nonarbitrary way. Beauchamp and Childress have offered the following guidelines for balancing conflicting principles:

- Good reasons can be offered to act on the overriding norm rather than on the infringed norm.
- The moral objective justifying the infringement has a realistic prospect of achievement.
- No morally preferable alternative actions are available.
- The lowest level of infringement, commensurate with achieving the primary goal of the action, has been selected.
- Any negative effects of the infringement have been minimized.
- All affected parties have been treated impartially (4).

As will be seen throughout this text, the principle of autonomy has come to occupy a central place in contemporary health care ethics and practice. For example, it provides an ethical grounding for the development of advance directives (see Chapter 8). Or again, it is now standard practice that patients give their "informed consent" to medical treatments and procedures and to various practices within a health care institution and, "since the mid-1970s, the primary justification advanced for requirements of informed consent has been to protect autonomous choice" (4). Or again, the HIPAA (Health Insurance Portability and Accountability Act) Privacy Rule imposes stringent administrative requirements on the collection, maintenance, transmission, use, and disclosure of individually identifiable health information (7). According to the U.S. Office for Civil Rights, the Privacy Rule "gives patients more control over their health information" and enables them "to make informed choices when seeking care and reimbursement for care based on how personal health information may be used" (8). From this perspective, the HIPAA privacy regulations are in line with the ethical emphasis on individual autonomy.

The emphasis currently being placed on patient autonomy is, at least in part, a reaction to the paternalistic way in which the health care professions were practiced at one time. The health care providers were the ones who made the treatment decisions, and the patient and family members tended to go along with what they said without raising questions. The emphasis on patient autonomy may also reflect the American emphasis on individualism (5, 9).

While no one is advocating a return to a purely paternalist approach on the part of health care providers, some concern is now being raised that the pendulum has swung too far in the other direction. There is concern that patient autonomy has gone too far and that some limits on it are in order. For example, some are arguing that a patient should not be entitled to receive medical treatments that are futile and that health care providers have the right to override patient wishes when futile treatments are wanted (see Chapter 7). Others offer a more radical criticism of the very concept of patient autonomy, maintaining that a focus on the patient alone is misguided (5).

Out of feminist work in ethics has come the *ethics of care*. This approach to ethics is described in the following way:

> . . . girls, being brought up by mothers, identify with them, while males must define themselves through separation from their mothers. . . . Thus while masculinity is defined by separation and threatened by intimacy, femininity is defined through attachment and threatened by separation; girls come to understand themselves as imbedded within a network of personal relationships. . . .
>
> The feminine voice in ethics attends to the particular other, thinks in terms of responsibilities to care for others, is sensitive to our interconnectedness, and strives to preserve relationships. It contrasts with the masculine voice, which speaks in terms of justice and rights, stresses consistency and principles, and emphasizes the autonomy of the individual and impartiality in one's dealings with others (10).

This feminist approach to ethics is "frequently described in terms of webs or networks" (5) and emphasizes "relationships and connections" rather than "isolated individuals" (5).

It has been claimed that the ethics of care is already part of the way we naturally reason in health care ethics:

> Looking at ethics committees, Sichel argues that a feminist ethics of caring is often part of the ethics committee's deliberations. She uses as an example the case of an incompetent elderly patient whose wishes are known but whose children disagree about what course to follow. She accurately notes that, although the committee will support following the patient's wishes, it will go to considerable lengths and spend considerable time in an attempt to obtain consensus about this course from all the children, believing that it has a duty to care about the family as well as the patient. It would appear that if the patient's wishes were the only important factor, the course of action desired by the patient should be followed immediately, rather than after the children have been persuaded to agree (5).

In sum, rather than focusing exclusively on what the patient wants (the principle of patient autonomy), the ethics of care directs us to attend to all the players in an ethical dilemma.

Consequentialist Theories

Consequentialist ethical theories, as the name indicates, judge rightness and wrongness of action on the basis of the consequences of action. The right action to perform is the one which, among the alternatives, has the best consequences overall. Or, if all the possible courses of action have negative consequences overall, the right action to perform is the one with the least bad consequences. Different consequentialist theories are generated by the range of consequences taken into account. An *ethical egoist* considers the consequences only for himself or herself as the agent of the action. The more popular (and plausible) theory of *utilitarianism* considers the consequences for everyone to be affected by the action, taking into account the impact on other people as well as the agent of the action (11).

Historically, utilitarianism was formulated by two British philosophers, Jeremy Bentham (12) and John Stuart Mill (13), in the eighteenth and nineteenth centuries. It is commonly known as the philosophy of "the greatest good for the greatest number" (14).

The classic utilitarianism of Bentham and Mill was hedonistic, judging consequences of actions in terms of pleasure and pain produced (12, 13).
As Mill states the theory:

The creed which accepts as the foundation of morals "utility" or the "greatest happiness principle" holds that actions are right in proportion as they tend to promote happiness; wrong as they tend to produce the reverse of happiness. By happiness is intended pleasure and the absence of pain; by unhappiness, pain and the privation of pleasure. (13)

Contemporary utilitarians are not necessarily hedonists (15). However, they still adhere to Mill's idea that we need to consider the consequences of actions not only for ourselves, but for everyone who will be affected by what we do:

. . . the happiness which forms the utilitarian standard of what is right in conduct is not the agent's own happiness but that of all concerned. As between his own happiness and that of others, utilitarianism requires him to be as strictly impartial as a disinterested and benevolent spectator. In the golden rule of Jesus of Nazareth, we read the complete spirit of the ethics of utility. "To do as you would be done by," and "to love your neighbor as yourself," constitute the ideal perfection of utilitarian morality (13).

The philosopher Carl Cohen gives an example of the application of utilitarianism to the controversial issue of the use of animals in biomedical research:

Those who claim to base their objection to the use of animals in biomedical research on the reckoning of net pleasures and pains produced make a second error . . . a cogent utilitarian calculation requires that we weigh all the consequences of the use, and of the nonuse, of animals in laboratory research. Critics relying . . . on animal rights may claim to ignore the beneficial results of such research, rights being trump cards to which interest and advantage must give way. But an argument that is explicitly framed in terms of interest and benefit for all over the long run must attend also to the disadvantageous consequences of not using animals in research, and to all the achievements attained and attainable only through their use. The sum of the benefits of their use is utterly beyond quantification. The elimination of horrible disease, the increase of longevity, the avoidance of great pain, the saving of lives, and the improvement of the quality of lives (for humans and for animals) achieved through research using animals is so incalculably great that the argument of these critics, systematically pursued, establishes not their conclusion but its reverse: to refrain from using animals in biomedical research is, on utilitarian grounds, morally wrong (16).

It is important to keep in mind that, for the utilitarian, no action is intrinsically right or wrong. Rightness and wrongness are determined entirely by consequences of actions.

Kant's Categorical Imperative

An ethical theory that makes moral judgments on the basis of considerations other than the consequences of actions is that of the eighteenth century German philosopher Immanuel Kant. Kant named his fundamental ethical principle the *categorical imperative*. He gave different formulations of the categorical imperative, stating his fundamental ethical principle in different ways. The two most famous formulations are the *universal law* formula, and the *end in itself* formula. It is the end in itself formula of the categorical imperative that has recently been used in dealing with issues in health care ethics.

Kant stated the end in itself formula in this way: "So act as to treat humanity, whether in thine own person or in that of any other, in every case as an end withal, never as a means only . . ." (17). This is an explanation of what he means:

> According to this formulation, rational creatures should always treat other rational creatures as ends in themselves and never as only means to ends. This formulation underscores Kant's belief that every human being has an inherent worth resulting from the sheer possession of rationality. We must always act in a way that respects this humanity in others and in ourselves. (11)

According to Kant, we act wrongly if we merely "use" another person to get something we want. We act rightly only if we treat human beings, both other people and ourselves, as beings having inherent, intrinsic worth. Kant's end in itself formula is sometimes referred to as a principle of "respect for persons" (18).

Suppose that a teenage girl is dying of cancer and that all known treatments have failed to help her. Her physicians suggest use of an experimental drug. The physicians do not believe that the drug will help this girl. In fact, they candidly tell her parents that she is likely to suffer from fever and vomiting if she takes it (which will increase her suffering as she dies). However, if she does take the drug, the physicians will gain information about how cancer patients tolerate it. This information will be valuable in using the drug in the future with other cancer patients who may be helped by it (19).

The parents of this teenage victim of cancer declined to have this experimental drug administered to their daughter (19). Kantian ethics would support their decision. The drug would not benefit their daughter. Rather, her suffering in taking the drug would simply be the means to benefit other people. Their daughter is a person with inherent worth and, as such, priority should be placed on making her death as peaceful and free of suffering as possible. She should not be "used" as a research guinea pig.

It should be noted that utilitarians and Kantians can come to different conclusions about the right thing to do in a particular case. A utilitarian would favor the administration of the experimental drug because of the good consequences overall. While the teenager will suffer, the negative value of her suffering will be outweighed by the good consequences for other people.

Ethics of Duty

Another dimension of our ethical discourse is talk about "duties," or interchangeably, about "obligations" (20). We speak of a duty to vote, a duty to take care of elderly parents, a duty to take care of our health, a duty to take care of the environment.

The twentieth century English philosopher W.D. Ross formulated an entire ethical theory based on the concept of duty (4, 20–22). Ross spoke of *prima facie* duties; that is, of duties "at first sight" or "other things being equal" (22). In other words, a prima facie duty "dictates what I should do when other relevant factors in a situation are not considered" (22). Ross claimed that the following prima facie duties are generally recognized on an intuitive basis:

1. Duties of fidelity: telling the truth, keeping promises.
2. Duties of reparation: righting the wrongs we have done to others.
3. Duties of gratitude: recognizing the services others have done for us.
4. Duties of justice: preventing a distribution of pleasure or happiness that is not in keeping with the merit of the people involved.
5. Duties of beneficence: helping to better the condition of other beings with respect to virtue, intelligence, or pleasure.
6. Duties of self-improvement: bettering ourselves with respect to virtue or intelligence.
7. Duties of nonmaleficence: avoiding or preventing an injury to others (22).

Ross makes a distinction between prima facie duties and our *actual duty* in a particular situation. In some cases, several prima facie duties may apply and be in conflict in what they tell us to do. This is reminiscent of what can happen with the theory of principlism described earlier. Ross offers two guidelines for determining our actual duty in such cases. First, in the case of two conflicting prima facie duties, he maintains that one's actual duty consists in the act that is in accord with the more stringent prima facie obligation. Further, when several prima facie duties are in conflict, he holds that one's actual duty is the act that has the greatest balance of prima facie rightness over prima facie wrongness. However, a weakness in Ross's theory is that he does not give us any concrete directions for determining when one duty is "more stringent" than another or for determining the "balance" of prima facie rightness over wrongness (22).

In spite of this weakness, it has been observed that Ross's theory is useful in a health care context in encouraging "each person responsible for patient care to reflect on the prima facie obligations that he or she has toward those people and to set aside one of those obligations only when morally certain that another obligation takes precedence" (22).

For example, suppose that a transplant surgeon detects signs of tissue rejection in a patient who has just had a kidney transplant. The surgeon is virtually certain that, within a week, the kidney will have to be surgically removed and the patient put on dialysis. However, the patient is suffering from postoperative depression and, if the patient is told right now that the transplant appears to be a failure, his depression may well become more severe. In turn, this could lead to a worsening of the patient's physical condition, maybe even to a degree that is life-threatening (23).

Relevant to this case is the duty of fidelity, which dictates that the physician should tell the patient the truth about his situation. On the other hand, the duty of nonmaleficence is also relevant, which dictates that the patient should not be told the truth because such knowledge might well cause him serious harm. Thus, the duties of fidelity and nonmaleficence are in conflict.

In this situation, the surgeon might decide that the duty of nonmaleficence takes precedence at the present time. The patient does not immediately have to be told of the impending need for surgery to remove the kidney and, by the time that need arises, his psychological condition may have improved (23).

Natural Law

The idea of a natural law goes back to Greek and Roman legal thought, where one finds this idea among Stoics and in the writings of Cicero. Natural law theory flourished in the high and late Middle Ages. In this period, the classic statement of natural law theory was given by Thomas Aquinas, but many other philosophers and theologians held it as well (24). Natural law theory continued into the early Modern period, being found in the writings of such philosophers as Thomas Hobbes (25) and John Locke (26). Among all the theories that go under the name of natural law, there is a common core of beliefs; namely, that the basic principles of morals and legislation are, in some sense or other, objective, accessible to reason, and, very importantly, based on human nature (24).

In its classic form as presented by Aquinas, natural law ethics holds that what is in accord with human nature is to be considered right, and what goes against human nature is to be considered wrong. More exactly, we find that human nature has certain properties. These properties entail that a human being ought to do acts *a, b,* and *c* and ought not to do acts *x, y,* and *z* (24). For example, we find that human beings have a natural inclination to self-preservation. What is in accord with self-preservation is right. It is right to exercise regularly in order to keep in shape physically since this promotes self-preservation. On the other hand, assisted suicide and euthanasia go against the natural inclination to self-preservation, and hence, are judged ethically wrong actions. Some natural law ethicists look not only at natural inclinations but also at goals or purposes embedded in human beings and activities in determining what is in accord with human nature (27).

Natural law has been used by the Catholic Church in evaluating assisted reproductive technologies. For example, the Catholic Church has used natural law reasoning to rule out the use of in vitro fertilization by husband and wife. What occurs naturally is that the act of sexual intercourse has two functions or goals. It is an expression of love between two people (unitive purpose) but it is also the means by which children are conceived (procreative purpose). Both of these purposes are found in the same act. It would be "unnatural" to separate the conception of a child from an interpersonal act of sexual intercourse. However, by fertilizing an ovum in a laboratory, this is precisely what in vitro fertilization does. Hence, according to natural law ethics, in vitro fertilization is to be judged ethically impermissible (28).

It should be noted that certain principles of relevance to health care ethics have also come out of the natural law tradition, such as the principle of double effect. Basically, this principle justifies taking a course of action that has two types of effects: one effect is perfectly good and is what is wanted, while the other effect is bad and is not wanted but may accompany the first (29). For example, among those opposed to abortion, the principle of double effect has been used to justify the removal of a cancerous uterus when a woman is pregnant. The desired effect is the removal of a diseased organ, which is a perfectly legitimate aim. In the case of pregnancy, however, removing the cancerous uterus will also mean the death of the fetus. The woman who is pregnant may not want to lose the child she is carrying, but this will be an unavoidable effect of removing the diseased organ (29).

In its fully developed form, the principle of double effect includes the following stipulations: the act itself must be morally good or neutral, only the good consequences of the act must be intended, the good effect must not be produced by means of the evil effect, and there must be some weighty reason for permitting the evil (30). For example, the act of removing a diseased organ, such as a cancerous uterus, is at least morally neutral and very possibly can be considered a morally good action. If a woman feels a loss because of the death of her child, it is clear that it is only the good consequence of removing a diseased organ which is intended by her, not the evil effect of the death of the child. If the cancerous uterus is removed with the fetus in it (rather than the fetus being killed before the removal of the uterus), then the evil effect of the death of the child is not the means of achieving the good effect. Finally, saving the life of the woman by removing a cancerous organ is certainly a weighty reason for permitting the evil of the death of her fetus.

Ethical Relativism vs. Ethical Objectivism

In discussing ethical theories and principles, a related issue that needs to be addressed is that of ethical relativism.

It is an undeniable fact that different groups of people—different societies, cultures, and subcultures—differ in their ethical judgments. For example, Hindus attribute a sacred status to cows, and consider it wrong to kill and eat them (31). On the other hand, raising cattle for food is a major industry in the United States. Some Islamic traditions require a woman to wear a burka, an outer garment that cloaks the entire body, in public. This is done for the sake of promoting modesty in dress and behavior in public (32). Mormon fundamentalist sects allow the practice of "plural marriage," a form of polygamy in which a man may have many wives. Mainline Mormons, on the other hand, practice monogamy (33). Or again, just consider the vigorous debates over abortion in the United States.

The fact of disagreement in ethical judgments has promoted the position known as *ethical relativism*. Ethical relativism denies that there are objectively true ethical standards that are valid for everyone everywhere. The relativist maintains that what is right and wrong varies among different cultures and societies (34). Thus, according to the relativist, euthanasia and physician aid-in-dying may be ethically right in one culture but wrong in another. In making this claim, the relativist is not speaking merely of what people may think is right or wrong, because people can make mistakes in their ethical judgments. Rather, the relativist is asserting that what in fact is right or wrong varies among different cultures and societies.

Ethical relativism is *not* itself an ethical theory or principle. Rather, it makes a claim *about* ethical theories and principles. It claims that no ethical theory or principle holds good for everyone everywhere. According to the relativist, utilitarianism may be an appropriate ethical theory for one society, but not for another. The principle of patient autonomy may be right for North Americans but not for Asians.

The West has sometimes suffered from *ethnocentrism*, the belief that its culture is inherently superior to other cultures (34). Such a view has been condemned "as a variety of prejudice tantamount to racism and sexism" (34). A reaction to ethnocentrism is a movement "not to judge others but to be tolerant of diversity" (34). Ethical relativism seems to fit with such an "attitude of tolerance toward other cultures" (34).

Some philosophers, however, have argued that ethical relativism has implications that go against common sense and common practice. These unacceptable implications are reasons for judging ethical relativism to be incorrect.

For one thing, ethical relativism prevents us from ever criticizing the practices of another society as evil:

> Suppose, a society waged war on its neighbors for the purpose of taking slaves. Or suppose a society was violently anti-Semitic, and its leaders set out to destroy the Jews. Cultural Relativism would preclude us from saying that either of these practices was wrong. We would not even be able to say that a society tolerant of Jews is *better* than the anti-Semitic society, for that would imply some sort of transcultural standard of comparison. The failure to condemn *these* practices does not seem "enlightened"; on the contrary, slavery and anti-Semitism seem wrong *wherever* they occur. Nevertheless, if we took Cultural Relativism seriously, we would have to admit that these social practices also are immune from criticism. (35)

These societal practices would be immune from criticism precisely because what is right and wrong is determined by the particular society.

Moreover, ethical relativism destroys our notion of social reform. For relativism "seems to entail that reformers are always (morally) wrong, because they go against the cultural tide" (34). However, "we normally feel just the opposite: that the reformer is the courageous innovator who is right, who has the truth, against the mindless majority" (34).

Further, ethical relativism destroys the notion of moral progress. This point can be illustrated by the changing status of women in society:

> Usually, we think that at least some changes in our society have been for the better . . . Throughout most of Western history the place of women in society was very narrowly circumscribed. They could not own property; they could not vote or hold political office; with a few exceptions, they were not permitted to have paying jobs; and generally they were under the almost absolute control of their husbands. Recently much of this has changed, and most people think of it as progress.
>
> If Cultural Relativism is correct, can we legitimately think of this as progress? Progress means replacing a way of doing things with a *better* way. But by what standard do we judge the new ways as better? If the old ways were in accordance with the social standards of their time, then Cultural Relativism would say it is a mistake to judge them by the standards of a different time. Eighteenth-century society was, in effect, a different society from the one we have now. To say that we have made progress implies a judgment that present-day society is better, and that is just the sort of transcultural judgment that, according to Cultural Relativism, is impermissible (35).

However, it does make sense to think that our society has made some moral progress. Because ethical relativism "says that these judgments make no sense," so the argument goes, "it cannot be right" (35).

According to ethical relativism, right and wrong are determined by a culture or society. This contention entails yet another problem because "one person may belong to several societies (subcultures) with different value emphases and arrangements of principles" (34). For example, "if Mary is a U.S. citizen and a member of the Roman Catholic Church, she is wrong (as a Catholic) if she chooses to have an abortion and not wrong (as a U.S. citizen) if she acts against the teaching of the Church on abortion" (34). According to relativism, just what is the ethically right thing for Mary to do?

In sum, there are serious problems with ethical relativism. The alternative view is ethical objectivism, the position that there are some ethical principles—at least, some basic or core ethical principles—that are valid for everyone everywhere (36). But then how does one account for the diversity of ethical judgments actually found in our world? Here is one explanation:

> Consider a culture in which people believe it is wrong to eat cows. This may even be a poor culture, in which there is not enough food; still, the cows

are not to be touched. Such a society would *appear* to have values very different from our own. But does it? We have not yet asked why these people will not eat cows. Suppose it is because they believe that after death the souls of humans inhabit the bodies of animals, especially cows, so that a cow may be someone's grandmother. Now do we want to say that their values are different from ours? No, the difference lies elsewhere. The difference is in our belief systems, not in our values. We agree that we shouldn't eat Grandma; we simply disagree about whether the cow is (or could be) Grandma. (35)

In other words, opponents of ethical relativism claim that different cultures and societies may share the same basic ethical principles and values but put these principles and values into practice in different ways because of different factual beliefs. Or again, the same principles and values may be put into practice in different ways because of different circumstances. For example, it has been suggested that Eskimos kill perfectly normal infants *not* because they have less affection for their children or less respect for human life than we do, but for reasons having to do with their lifestyle and survival. Eskimo mothers will nurse their children for 4 years, which places limits on the number of infants that one mother can sustain. In addition, Eskimos are nomadic since they are unable to farm, and a mother can carry only one baby as she travels (35).

While flaws are apparent in ethical relativism, can anything be said positively in favor of ethical objectivism? It has been argued that "there are some moral rules that all societies will have in common, because those rules are necessary for society to exist" (35). A prohibition against lying is given as one example:

Imagine what it would be like for a society to place no value at all on truth telling. When one person spoke to another, there would be no presumption at all that he was telling the truth—for he could just as easily be speaking falsely. Within that society, there would be no reason to pay attention to what anyone says. (I ask you what time it is, and you say "four o'clock." But there is no presumption that you are speaking truly; you could just as easily have said the first thing that came into your head. So, I have no reason to pay attention to your answer—in fact, there was no point in my asking you in the first place!) Communication would then be extremely difficult, if not impossible. And because complex societies cannot exist without regular communication among their members, society would become impossible. It follows that in any complex society there *must* be a presumption in favor of truthfulness (35).

The prohibition against murder is given as another example of a rule needed for a society to survive (35). One philosopher has developed the following list of core moral principles binding on all human beings:

1. It is morally wrong to torture people for the fun of it.
2. Do not kill innocent people.
3. Do not cause pain or suffering except when a higher duty prescribes it.
4. Do not commit rape.
5. Keep your promises and contracts.
6. Do not deprive another person of his or her freedom.
7. Do justice, treating equals equally and unequals unequally.
8. Tell the truth.
9. Help other people.
10. Obey just laws (34).

Among these allegedly common moral principles, [2], [3], [5], [7], [8], and [9] have definite implications for the field of health care.

References

1. Diane E. Hoffmann, Philip Boyle, and Steven A. Levenson, *Handbook for Nursing Home Ethics Committees* (Washington, DC: American Association of Homes and Services for the Aging, 1995).
2. Patrick Norris, OP, "The McCaughey Septuplets: All's Well that Ends Well?" *Health Care Ethics USA* (Spring 1998): 6–7.
3. Michael D. Lemonick, "It's a Miracle," *Time* (December 1, 1997): 34–39.
4. Tom L. Beauchamp and James F. Childress, *Principles of Biomedical Ethics*, 6th ed. (New York: Oxford, 2009).
5. Judith Wilson Ross, John W. Glaser, Dorothy Rasinki-Gregory, Joan McIver Gibson, and Corrine Bayley, *Health Care Ethics Committees The Next Generation* (Chicago: American Hospital Publishing, 1993).
6. Ronald Munson, "Principles of Distributive Justice" in Ronald Munson (ed.), *Intervention and Reflection Basic Issues in Medical Ethics*, 8th ed. (Belmont, CA: Thomson Wadsworth, 2008).
7. Maureen Weaver, Jeanette C. Schreiber, Michelle Wilcox DeBarge, Catherine P. Baatz, Wiggin band Dana, LLP, *The HIPAA Handbook Implementing the Federal Privacy Rule in the Long-Term Care Setting* (Washington, DC: American Association of Homes and Services for the Aging, 2001).

8. Office of Civil Rights, *Standards for Privacy of Individually Identifiable Health Information,* http://www.hhs.gov/ocr/hipaa/finalmaster.html. Accessed 2002.

9. Robert N. Bellah, Richard Madsen, William M. Sullivan, Ann Swidler, and Steven M. Tipton, *Habits of the Heart* (New York: Harper & Row, 1985).

10. Celia Wolf-Devine, "Abortion and the 'Feminine Voice,'" *Public Affairs Quarterly* 3/3 (July 1989): 81–97.

11. William H. Shaw, "Normative Theories of Ethics" in William H. Shaw (ed.), *Social and Personal Ethics,* 2nd ed. (Belmont, CA: Wadsworth, 1996).

12. Jeremy Bentham, *An Introduction to the Principles of Morals and Legislation in The Utilitarians* (Garden City, NY: Anchor/Doubleday, 1973).

13. John Stuart Mill, *Utilitarianism* (Indianapolis: Bobbs-Merrill, 1957).

14. Julie Driver, "The History of Utilitarianism," *The Stanford Encyclopedia of Philosophy* (Winter 2014 edition). http://plato.stanford.edu/archive/win2014/entries/utilitarianism-history. Accessed May 2016.

15. *Does the End Justify the Means?* Intelecom DVD.

16. Carl Cohen, "The Case Against Animal Rights," in Louis J. Pojman and Lewis Vaughn (eds.), *The Moral Life An Introductory Reader in Ethics and Literature,* 3rd ed. (New York: Oxford University Press, 2007).

17. Immanuel Kant, *The Foundations of the Metaphysics of Morals,* trans. T.K. Abbott in William H. Shaw (ed.), *Social and Personal Ethics,* 2nd ed. (Belmont, CA: Wadsworth, 1996).

18. Elizabeth S. Anderson, "Is Women's Labor a Commodity?" *Philosophy and Public Affairs* 19/1 (Winter 1990): 71–87, 90–92.

19. *Human Experiments: The Price of Knowledge?* KCTS/Seattle, 1980, video.

20. William K. Frankena, *Ethics,* 2nd ed. (Englewood Cliffs, NJ: Prentice-Hall, 1973).

21. W.D. Ross, *The Right and the Good* (Oxford: Oxford University Press, 1930).

22. "Ross's Ethics" in Ronald Munson (ed.), *Intervention and Reflection: Basic Issues in Medical Ethics,* 8th ed. (Belmont, CA: Thomson Wadsworth, 2008).

23. "Truth Telling in Medicine" in Ronald Munson (ed.), *Intervention and Reflection: Basic Issues in Medical Ethics,* 8th ed. (Belmont, CA: Thomson Wadsworth, 2008).

24. D.J. O'Connor, *Aquinas and Natural Law* (London: Macmillan, 1967).

25. Thomas Hobbes, *Leviathan* (New York: E.P. Dutton, 1950).

26. John Locke, *Essays on the Law of Nature,* trans. W. von Leyden (Oxford: Clarendon, 1965).

27. Jacques Maritain, *Natural Law: Reflections on Theory and Practice* (South Bend, IN: St. Augustine's Press, 2001).

28. Vatican Congregation for the Doctrine of the Faith, *Instruction on Respect for Human Life in its Origin and On the Dignity of Procreation* (Washington, DC: United States Catholic Conference, 1987).

29. Orville N. Griese, *Catholic Identity in Health Care: Principles and Practice* (Braintree, MA: Pope John Center, 1987).

30. President's Commission for the Study of Ethical Problems in Medicine and Biomedical and Behavioral Research, *Deciding to Forego Life-Sustaining Treatment* (1983; reprint New York: Concern for Dying).

31. Religionfacts, *The Cow in Hinduism.* http://www.religionfacts.com/hinduism /things/cow.htm. Accessed May 2016.

32. Wikipedia, s.v. Burqa. http://en.wikipedia.org/wiki/Burqa. Accessed April 2009.

33. Wikipedia, s.v. Mormon fundamentalism. http://en.wikipedia.org/wiki/ Morman _Fundamentalism. Accessed May 2016.

34. Louis Pojman, "Ethical Relativism versus Ethical Objectivism," in Louis P. Pojman (ed.), *Introduction to Philosophy: Classical and Contemporary Readings* (Belmont, CA: Wadsworth, 1991).

35. James Rachels, "The Challenge of Cultural Relativism," in Joel Feinberg (ed.), *Reason and Responsibility: Readings in Some Basic Problems of Philosophy*, 9th ed. (Belmont, CA: Wadsworth, 1996).

36. Louis Pojman, "A Critique of Ethical Relativism," in Louis Pojman (ed.), *Ethical Theory Classical and Contemporary Readings*, 3rd ed. (Belmont, CA: Wadsworth, 1998).

Chapter 2

Ethics Committees: A Resource for Resolving Ethical Dilemmas

Many of the most puzzling questions faced today by health care providers and by patients and their families are not exclusively medical in character, but involve individual and institutional values. Ethics committees raise consciousness about the moral dimensions of health care decision making and provide a forum for working through difficult ethical problems.

While ethics committees began in the acute care, hospital setting, they have expanded to long-term care facilities and other types of health care services. Initially, ethics committees focused on issues in *clinical practice*. They discussed, for example, when it is permissible to withhold or withdraw life-sustaining treatments. Some committees have expanded the scope of their activity to include *organizational ethics*, considering administrative, financial, and human resource questions (1). In fact, some facilities have established separate clinical and organizational ethics committees. In this book, we focus on the work of ethics committees in a clinical context.

Functions of an Ethics Committee

An ethics committee typically has three main functions: education, the development and review of institutional policies and guidelines, and case consultation.

One of the primary functions of an ethics committee is providing education on issues related to health care ethics. This includes education of the committee members themselves, who come from a variety of professional backgrounds. It also includes continuing education and in-service programs for health care providers within the facility. In addition, ethics committees engage in community education, developing programming for the general public.

Second, ethics committees are involved in developing and reviewing policies and guidelines for the facility that have an ethical dimension. For example, an ethics committee may assist in developing a policy on futile medical treatment to be sent to the facility's medical staff, nursing staff and/or board for approval. Or the committee may be asked to review and revise a policy that is already in place on Do-Not-Resuscitate orders or on the use of restraints.

Third, an ethics committee is typically available for consultation with patients, family members, and health care providers about difficult ethical dilemmas they face. This committee activity will later be described at length.

The Make-Up of an Ethics Committee

Ethics committees usually comprise between twelve and fifteen members. The membership is multidisciplinary, representing various types of work in health care and various professions. The committee is not necessarily composed entirely of employees of the facility; it may include some individuals from within the community the facility serves.

An ethics committee, whether at a hospital or a long-term care facility, typically includes representation from the following groups:

- board of trustees;
- administration;
- medical staff (physicians);
- nursing staff;
- clergy/pastoral care staff;
- social workers;

- attorneys;
- ethicists;
- patient advocates (for example, parent of a disabled child, resident of a senior living facility).

However, this does not preclude membership by other types of health care professionals. Consistent with the concept of an integrated community health care system, an ethics committee may also include representatives from such areas as pharmacy, allied health, hospice services, home health care, adult day care, and assisted living services.

Many ethics committees serve just one particular facility. However, a number of facilities in a particular geographical area will sometimes join together to establish a regional ethics committee serving all the participating facilities. Some ethics committees meet monthly, others meet bi-monthly, and yet others meet only quarterly.

Ethics Consultation

Patients and family members can discuss the ethical dimensions of treatment decisions with their health care providers or with pastoral care staff. Health care providers can talk with coworkers. However, a time may come when patients, family, or health care providers feel that they have reached the limits of their own abilities to address an ethical issue. In such cases, an ethics consult may be a helpful resource.

An *ethics consult* is a meeting with members of the ethics committee to work through difficult issues in patient care from the point of view of moral rightness and wrongness. Sometimes the whole ethics committee will be involved, sometimes a subcommittee of it.

An ethics consult may

- provide information about ethical principles relevant to the case under discussion;
- clarify what the caregiving options are;
- provide information about similar cases;
- provide information about relevant policies of the facility;
- result in recommendations that are advisory in nature.

Ethics consultation services are not intended to replace the normal lines of communication among health care providers, patients, and families. But an ethics consult may be helpful when

- a patient, family member, or health care provider wants help in "talking through" ethical issues involved in patient care;
- there is a serious ethical disagreement between health care providers, among family members, between health care providers and the patient, or between health care providers and family members;
- ethically, the case is unusual, unprecedented, or very complex;
- a patient, family member, or health care provider would like to have the benefit of other perspectives in working through an ethical problem.

Any recommendations made by the consultants are purely advisory in nature. Patients, family members, and health care providers remain responsible for making their own decisions.

A notation that an ethics consult has taken place may be put into the patient's medical record. Ethics consults are treated as confidential. They may subsequently be discussed by the members of the ethics committee, but with appropriate safeguards for maintaining confidentiality (2).

The Emergence of Bioethics Mediation

Perhaps the most challenging ethics consults involve situations of conflict. In response, ethics consultants have attempted to bring into their work the skills and procedures traditionally associated with mediation (3). Thus, the practice of bioethics mediation has evolved.

While traditional ethics consults may well be conducted by a group of persons, formal bioethics mediation is conducted by an individual. The mediator must have both subject-matter expertise in bioethics and expertise in communication skills (3, 4). The goal of bioethics mediation has been described as reaching a "principled resolution" to the conflict (3, 4), which is "a clinical plan of action agreed upon by relevant stakeholders and chosen from among multiple morally permissible options that fall within the spectrum of acceptable clinical, ethical, and legal outcomes" (3). In other words, bioethics mediation involves determining the parameters set for the case by clinical, ethical, and legal considerations; determining what courses of action (in the plural) fall within these parameters; and achieving agreement among the relevant stakeholders on one of those courses of action.

The increasing importance of bioethics mediation is indicated by the fact that the University of Pennsylvania is offering a Certificate in Clinical Ethics Mediation as an adjunct to its Master of Bioethics Degree (5).

References

1. Judith Wilson Ross, et al., *Health Care Ethics Committees The Next Generation* (Chicago: American Hospital Publishing, 1993).
2. The information on ethics consultation is adapted from brochures prepared by the Clinical Ethics Committee of Mercy Medical Center, Dubuque, Iowa and the Medical Ethics Committee of the University of Nebraska Medical Center.
3. Nancy Neveloff Dubler, "A 'Principled Resolution': The Fulcrum of Bioethics Mediation," *Law and Contemporary Problems* 74/177 (Summer 2011): 177–200.
4. Nancy Neveloff Dubler and Carol B. Liebman, *Bioethics Mediation A Guide to Shaping Shared Solutions,* revised and expanded ed. (Nashville: Vanderbilt University Press, 2011).
5. University of Pennsylvania Department of Medical Ethics and Health Policy, *Clinical Ethics Mediation.* http://medicalethics.med.upenn.edu/education/master-of-bioethics-mbe/clinical-ethics-mediation. Accessed March 2016.

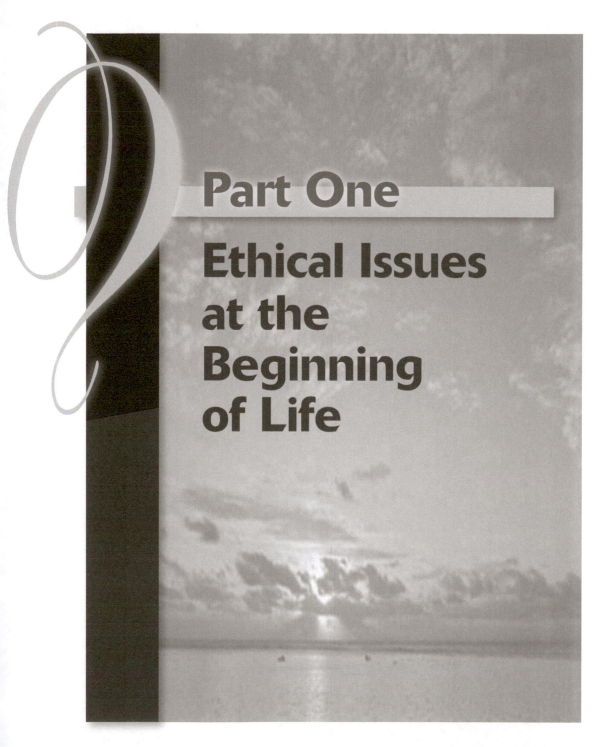

Part One

Ethical Issues at the Beginning of Life

Chapter 3

The Abortion Debate

Ever since the *Roe v. Wade* decision of the U.S. Supreme Court in 1973 legalizing the practice of abortion, abortion has been one of the most divisive issues in American society. People regularly categorize themselves as being either "pro-choice" or "pro-life."

Abortion may be defined as "the termination of a pregnancy with resulting death of the human fetus" (1). So defined, the term abortion is a generic term covering a number of different events and procedures. A distinction can be made between *spontaneous abortion*, which is another name for a miscarriage, and *induced* or *procured abortion*, which is caused by human action. Within the category of induced or procured abortions, a distinction can be made between *indirect* and *direct abortions*. An indirect abortion occurs when the direct, immediate purpose of the procedure is to treat the mother for a threatening pathology, but the death of the fetus is also an inevitable result (which would have been avoided if possible). An example of an indirect abortion is surgery to remove a cancerous uterus when a woman is pregnant. On the other hand, a direct abortion occurs when the direct, immediate purpose of the procedure is to destroy the human fetus or to expel it when it is not viable (1). Ethically, what is controversial is the practice of direct abortion, and it is this type of abortion that will be the focus of the present chapter. When the term "abortion" is used in this chapter, it will be understood as referring to "direct abortion."

Three different positions have been taken on the morality of abortion. First, there is the position of *abortion on demand,* which is the view that abortion is permissible at any time during a pregnancy for any reason whatever. A second position would allow *abortion in a limited number of cases;* for example, in cases of rape or incest, or when the fetus is suffering from a severe abnormality, or when the pregnancy threatens the well-being (physical or psychological) of the mother. The third position is that *abortion is never permissible.*

In this chapter, you will learn about:

■   common arguments for and against the ethical permissibility of abortion;
■   the controversy about when human life begins;
■   selective abortion in the case of fetal abnormality;
■   abortion in the case of rape.

Case Study

Connie and Roger Young are in their mid-thirties and have been married for eleven years. They have two children, Julie, 8, and Melissa 6. Although Melisssa is a special needs child, Connie has been able to resume teaching full-time, something she enjoys and finds self-fulfilling. Roger respects Connie's desire to pursue her own career. Besides, they can use the second income.

Barbara Cullen works as a speech and hearing therapist in the school system in which Connie teaches. Barbara and Connie have been good friends for some time. Lately, Barbara can tell that Connie has been agitated and upset.

One day when they are having lunch together, Barbara asks Connie what is wrong. Connie confesses that she has recently learned that she is pregnant—unexpectedly and unintentionally. She and Roger had decided they would have only the two children—no more. She had been using contraceptives for birth control, but obviously it didn't provide 100 percent protection. Roger, she says, has been trying to take a positive attitude toward having another child. Indeed, he has joked that maybe this time they will have the son he has always wanted!

Connie, on the other hand, is very concerned about what the birth of another child will do to her ability to provide Melissa with the extra attention that she needs and to her own developing teaching career. Further, having another child will put a strain on the family's financial resources, and she doubts that this is really fair to the welfare of the children they already have. Connie has told Roger that she feels she has to have an abortion. Roger, she tells Barbara, didn't like that at all.

Barbara has befriended some of the girls at school who have become pregnant, and tried to encourage them to think about and work through some of the issues—including ethical issues—surrounding abortion before they rush into having one. She wonders if she should take the same approach with her coworker Connie.

■ ■ ■

Common Arguments For and Against the Permissibility of Abortion

It has been reported that "the most common reason for seeking an abortion" is "not rape, incest, or concern for the life of the mother" but that "the circumstances of the pregnancy are not felt to be right, not right for the mother and not right for the one to be born" (2). These circumstances can include "broken families, drug abuse, crushing poverty, abusive relationships, incomplete education, fear of public humiliation, antagonistic partners and failed love" (2). In the hypothetical case of Connie Young, the circumstances making her feel that this pregnancy is not right are the welfare of the children she already has in terms of caregiving responsibilities and financial support, and her own welfare in terms of career fulfillment.

Personalizing common arguments in the abortion debate to the case of Connie Young, the following considerations might be brought forward in support of Connie's desire to have an abortion:

■ Connie will have to bear the risk and burden of pregnancy, delivery, and child care. It will be extremely difficult for her to undergo this unless it is her choice to do so (1).

- Connie has the right to a normal sex life, on which her marriage and the care of her other children also depend. Since artificial contraception does not give her complete control over pregnancy, she has the right to use abortion as a last resort (1).
- Connie has the right to control what happens to her body because it is her property. If a pregnancy occurs unintentionally and accidentally, the fetus can be compared to a trespasser on the woman's property who has no right to the use of her body (3).
- For Connie to bear an unwanted child will be a disaster for the child as well as for Connie. No matter how hard she may try, Connie may not be able to provide the child with the kind of atmosphere the child needs psychologically, and may even engage in child neglect or abuse (1).

On the other hand, the following arguments might be offered against Connie having an abortion:

- While continuing with the pregnancy may cause certain hardships for Connie, these hardships are not as severe as what the fetus suffers through abortion, namely, the complete loss of life. The fetus's right to life takes precedence over the avoidance of hardships for Connie (1).
- Everyone should realize that no method of birth control, other than abstinence, is 100 percent effective. By voluntarily engaging in sexual relations, Connie has given the fetus the right to use her body.
- Even if a woman's body is her property, this does not give her any right to kill a fetus within her body. In general, ownership of property does not give one the right to kill innocent people who are on, or even trespassing on, one's property. In fact, a property owner can be held responsible if people injure themselves while on his property (4).
- By having an abortion, Connie is guilty of taking an innocent human life.
- Having an abortion is not likely to relieve Connie of stress and give her peace of mind. Women who have abortions may later experience psychological repercussions for which they may have to seek counseling.
- As partly responsible for its existence, Roger also has rights concerning what is done with the fetus. If she proceeds with having an abortion contrary to Roger's wishes, Connie is ignoring and violating Roger's rights as a father.

The claim that abortion is wrong because it is an act of killing a human being is a major argument in the abortion debate. It deserves special attention.

The Controversy about the Beginning of Human Life

More formally stated, the argument at issue is this: Killing an innocent human being is ethically wrong; because abortion takes the life of an innocent human being, abortion must be considered ethically wrong.

The first premise of this argument, "Killing an innocent human being is ethically wrong," contains a qualification about "innocence." This qualification is meant to establish a distinction from the case of capital punishment in which an evildoer is killed. The second premise of the argument, "Abortion takes the life of an innocent human being," assumes that the fetus is a human being. This, in turn, raises the question of exactly when human life begins.

In *Roe v. Wade*, the 1973 U.S. Supreme Court decision legalizing abortion, the Court saw viability as the critical time in the pregnancy, after which there might be governmental regulation and even prohibition of abortion (5). Viability is the time at which a fetus can be removed from the mother's womb and live apart from her, perhaps with some technological assistance (5). At viability, the fetus has existence independent of the mother, and this is the reason it is taken as the beginning of an individual human life (2).

However, viability is not an absolutely fixed point, and this poses a problem for selecting it as the beginning of a human life. For one thing, the time of viability depends on the state of our technology. At the time of the *Roe v. Wade* decision in 1973, viability was placed at 28 weeks (6). However, by the 1980s, advances in neonatal care made 24 weeks the generally accepted dividing line (6). Indeed, "the perfection of artificial incubation may make the fetus viable at any time" (7). Moreover, mere length of life of the fetus is not an exact measure of viability.

> Perinatologists (specialists in newborns) say that too many factors are involved in determining viability to make reliable generalizations about which fetuses will live and which will die at any given stage of development. In addition to characteristics such as a fetus's weight and the developmental stage of the organs, factors like the health of the mother, her socioeconomic status, and her access to health care also play a role. So do the race and the gender of the fetus. In development, a white fetus generally lags a week behind an African American one of the same age, and a male fetus lags the same amount behind a female (8).

In sum, "if viability is the norm, the standard would vary with race and with many individual circumstances" (7). And if there is so much variability in viability, then viability does not seem to provide a secure basis for determining the time when human life begins.

Others push the beginning of human life back to the time of conception/ fertilization. Within this camp, some see a human being coming into existence as soon as the sperm has entered and united with the ovum; others see syngamy as the definitive point, when the nuclei of the ovum and the sperm have fused to form a new, single nucleus with a complete set of chromosomes (1, 9). The following biological facts about the embryo are cited to support classifying it as a human being from the time of conception/fertilization:

> First, the embryo is from the start distinct from any cell of the mother or of the father. This is clear because it is growing in its own distinct direction. Its growth is internally directed to its own survival and maturation. Second, the embryo is human: it has the genetic makeup characteristic of human beings. Third, and most important, the embryo is a complete or whole organism, though immature. The human embryo, from conception onwards, is fully programmed and has the active disposition to use that information to develop himself or herself to the mature stage of a human being, and, unless prevented by disease or violence, will actually do so. . . . None of the changes that occur to the embryo after fertilization, for as long as he or she survives, generates a new direction of growth. . . . Rather, all of the changes . . . either facilitate or retard the internally directed growth of this determinate and enduring individual (9).

Thus it is asserted that "a human embryo is not something different in kind from a human being, like a rock, or a potato, or a rhinoceros" (9). Rather, "a human embryo is a whole living member of the species Homo sapiens in the earliest stage of his or her natural development" (9).

One challenge to regarding conception/fertilization as the beginning of human life is found in our criteria for determining death. The irreversible cessation of brain activity is one of the accepted criteria of death (10). Therefore, by symmetry, should not the beginning of brain activity be taken as the beginning of human life? (2). Brain activity usually becomes detectable in the fetus during the eighth week, and the brain structure is complete at twelve weeks (9, 11).

One response to this challenge has been to point out a disanalogy between the case of brain death and the status of the embryo or fetus. After brain death has occurred, "a human being no longer will function as a person in the future" (2). It is "this lack of potentiality" that "leads to the determination of death" (2).

The case is different "if the brain is only temporarily not functioning properly, and the human being will be able to flourish in the future" (2). In this case, brain death has not taken place (2) and the person is not considered "not alive." Thus the potentiality for brain function is critical, and this exists in the embryo or fetus. With the embryo or fetus, the lack of brain function "is not permanent but only temporary due to a lack of maturity" (2). Thus, the status of the embryo or fetus is like "being in a temporary coma from which someone will entirely recover, rather than being brain dead" (2).

Those espousing the position that human life begins at the time of conception/fertilization have also contended that what is needed for human life to exist is "self-directed integral organic functioning" (9). In the case of human beings who have matured to the point at which the brain performs that role, brain death is recognized as the end of life because the irreversible cessation of brain functioning destroys that capacity (9). However, the embryo clearly exhibits self-directed integral organic functioning although this capability is achieved through other physiological factors than the brain (9).

Several biological facts about human reproduction are also brought forward against regarding conception/fertilization as the beginning point of a particular human life: twinning, embryo fusion, and natural wastage.

During the first 2 weeks after conception/fertilization, the embryo can split to form identical (monozygotic) twins, or even triplets or higher order multiples (12). This possibility provides evidence that "the early embryo is not yet one human being, but a community of possibly different individuals held together by a gelatinous membrane" (12). Moreover, it sometimes happens that "separate and genetically distinct embryos (which might have gone on to become fraternal twins) fuse during early development to form a single human being" (12). Hence, until the time for twinning and embryo recombination has passed, we do not know how many human beings are actually present. And until we know how many individuals are present, how can we speak of the beginning of their human life? Thus the phenomena of twinning and embryo fusion have led some to conclude that biological individuality is not established until the time of gastrulation, which begins at 2 weeks of gestational age (12).

On the other hand, it has been argued that being an "individual" does not require indivisibility (2). For example, a flatworm can be divided to produce two whole flatworms but it is not thought that, prior to the division, the original flatworm was not a unique individual (9). Similarly, amoeba can divide (13) and some plants have cells that can give rise to further plants (2), but in neither case do we deny the individuality of the entity prior to division. Thus the same should hold true in our thinking about the human embryo (9).

That the embryo is an individual life prior to twinning has also been defended on biological grounds:

> . . . in twinning, either the first embryo dies and gives rise to two others, or the first embryo continues to live and a second embryo is generated upon the splitting of the first one. We think the latter alternative is more likely, that twinning is . . . a type of asexual reproduction in which the second embryo is reproduced asexually. For although monozygotic twinning *can* occur at the two-cell stage, most monozygotic twinning (at least two-thirds) occurs between days 5 and 9. In those cases, the growth trajectory of the original embryo continues, though the separation of some of the cells from the inner cell mass generates another embryo, with a distinct development trajectory. (14)
>
> . . . the clearest evidence that the embryo in the first two weeks is not a mere mass of cells but is a unitary organism is this: if the individual cells within the embryo before twinning were each independent of the others, there would be no reason why each would not regularly develop on its own. Instead, these allegedly independent, noncommunicating cells regularly function together to develop into a single, more mature member of the human species. This fact shows that interaction is taking place between the cells from the very beginning . . . restraining them from individually developing as whole organisms and directing each of them to function as a relevant part of a single, whole organism continuous with the zygote. (15)

In sum, it is argued that the embryo, prior to any twinning, is an "individual" because of two biological facts. First, the process of twinning represents a process of asexual reproduction from the original embryo. Second, the individual cells within the embryo do not regularly go off on their own to form a complete human being but regularly function together to produce a single human being. This shows that they are not completely independent of each other but are interacting as part of a unitary organism (15).

The frequency of embryo fusion within the human population has not been precisely determined (12). Nevertheless, this phenomenon, however rare, does seem to pose a challenge to determining when human life begins. Experience teaches that two distinct human beings do not fuse into one. Since two embryos can fuse into one, this is taken as evidence that human embryos are not human individuals (2).

In response, philosophers have engaged in thought experiments to determine whether it makes sense conceptually for two human beings to fuse into one. Indeed, possible scenarios have been drawn from the media. For example, in the movie *All of Me* Lily Tomlin dies and ends up in the body of Steve Martin. This results in male and female psyches existing simultaneously in Steve Martin's body (2). Perhaps an even better example for our purposes comes from the Star Trek series, in which a transporter "can break down the molecular structure of a human being in one place and then reassemble the person in a new place" (2). In one episode of the series, "a transporter malfunctions turning two characters, Tuvok and Neelix, into a new combination, 'Tuvix,' a being not identical to either" (2). While we can wonder about the *identity* of the fused human being with respect to its antecedents, it is clear that two persons were present before the fusion (2). Similarly, two embryos that fuse could still have the status of being human beings from the time of conception/fertilization.

Natural wastage is another biological fact that has been seen to cast doubt on conception/fertilization as the beginning of human life:

> Reproductive embryologists report that human embryos have a very high natural rate of mortality during the first few weeks of development. Estimates vary greatly, but some studies suggest that in normal healthy women, between two-thirds and three-quarters of all fertilized eggs do not go on to implant in the womb. Some of this embryonic loss results from complex biological processes that screen embryos for genetic or chromosomal abnormalities. Embryos that fail to pass this test are sloughed off as a late menstrual period, often without any awareness on the woman's part that she was pregnant. . . . In view of this high rate of embryonic loss, do we truly want to bestow much moral significance on an entity with which nature is so wasteful? (12)

In reply, it has been pointed out that, since a number of these unsuccessful pregnancies are actually due to chromosomal defects, "it seems plausible to infer that in some cases, these defects are so significant that a human embryo probably failed to form" (9). In other words, "in some, and perhaps many cases, what is lost is not an embryo but a nonembryonic entity resulting from defects in the fertilization process" (9; see also 16). Further, even if embryos properly speaking are being lost, it has been noted that for centuries the rate of infant mortality throughout the world was greater than 50 percent, but this death rate did not disqualify the infants in question from having the status of a human being (2).

As noted in the *Roe v. Wade* decision, "those trained in the respective disciplines of medicine, philosophy, and theology" have not yet been able to "arrive at any consensus" about exactly when human life begins (5). However, it might be argued that, even if the embryo or fetus is not human until some point in development later than conception/fertilization, it is still the case that there is the *potential* for human life from the time of conception/fertilization. This potential for human life, it might be claimed, makes the developing embryo and fetus different from a mere clump of cells, and entitles its life to be protected.

Human Being vs. Human Person

Another twist in the abortion debate is to acknowledge that an embryo is a human being, but to make a distinction between a "human being" and a "human person" with the accompanying claim that it is only human "persons" who have rights, including a right to life (9). Characteristics that have been suggested as constituting "persons" include self-consciousness (of oneself as existing over time), a capacity to act on reasons, a capacity to communicate with others using a language, a capacity to act freely, and rationality (17). The claim is that, according to this standard, embryos and fetuses do not display the requisite cognitive characteristics to qualify as human "persons" and hence cannot be accorded a "right to life."

Several arguments have been offered against the plausibility of this position. First, proponents of this view "do not wish . . . to exclude from the status of 'persons' human beings who are asleep or who are in reversible comas" (9), so that the cognitive abilities in question must be construed as a "capacity or potentiality of some sort" (9). In other words, "sleeping or reversibly comatose human beings *are* persons because they have the potentiality or capacity for higher mental functions" (9). However, "human embryos and fetuses also possess, albeit in radical form, a capacity or potentiality for such mental functions" (9). Thus embryos and fetuses cannot be disqualified from the status of being human "persons."

Moreover, a developing human being does not display the cognitive characteristics in question until sometime after birth. For example, "a six-week-old baby lacks the immediately or even nearly immediately exercisable capacity to perform characteristically human mental functions" (9). Hence, "if full moral respect were due only to those who possess a nearly immediately exercisable capacity for characteristically human mental functions, it would follow that six-week-old infants do not deserve full moral respect" (9). And thus, "if abortion were morally acceptable on the grounds that the human embryo or fetus lacks such a capacity for characteristically human mental functions, then one would be logically committed to the view that, subject to parental approval, human infants could be disposed of as well" (9). To reach such a conclusion seems absurd.

Case Study

Anita and Sheila are sisters who have always been especially close. In fact, they married brothers, Robert and Allen. Anita got married first, followed bySheila two years later. Both love children and have always wanted to have three or four each.

However, when Sheila becomes pregnant, she decides to have the health of her fetus checked through prenatal diagnosis. This is because her sister Anita has already given birth to a son with cystic fibrosis, an inheritable genetic disorder. An ultrasound reveals that Sheila is carrying twins. Amniocentesis gives her the bad news that both of her babies have cystic fibrosis.

Cystic fibrosis (CF) causes the body to produce thick, sticky mucus that clogs the lungs and leads to life-threatening infections. Because of this, therapy must be done with children with CF several times a day. Occasionally, they require hospitalization. There is currently no cure for cystic fibrosis. Some people with CF live into their thirties, but some die at a much younger age.

More than once Anita has telephoned Sheila crying because of the strains of caregiving. Because of her son's needs, Anita has had to give up her teaching job and feels confined to her home. Because of her sister's experience, Sheila is aware of the time demands of caring for a CF child, and the emotional strain of worrying about the child's future and of having to face the possibility of the child's death. Having the responsibility of one CF child is enough, but having two such children to care for is more than Sheila thinks she can deal with.

Cystic fibrosis is a recessive genetic disorder. Although Sheila and her husband themselves do not have CF, they must both be carriers of the gene for CF in order to have a child affected by cystic fibrosis. For each pregnancy there is a 25 percent chance of conceiving a child affected by CF, and a 75 percent chance of conceiving a child who will not be affected by this genetic disorder. Sheila talks with her husband about aborting the two fetuses with CF she is carrying, and starting another pregnancy in the hope of conceiving a healthy child. After all, she thinks, bad luck can't be with them forever!

■ ■ ■

Selective Abortion for Fetal Abnormalities

What is at issue in the case of Sheila's pregnancy is known as "selective abortion." It is not the case that an abortion is performed because no child is wanted. Rather, an abortion is performed only to prevent the birth of a particular kind of child; in this case, a child with a genetic disease.

As well as the arguments used to justify abortion in general, some special considerations are brought forward in support of the selective abortion of fetuses with abnormalities:

- *Aborting abnormal fetuses prevents suffering for the family.* Parents encounter rough spots in raising any child, but the strains are increased in caring for a child suffering from a serious disease. The strains are not only financial, but also emotional (18).
- *Aborting an abnormal fetus prevents suffering for the child himself or herself.* Because of the suffering the disease would bring the child, giving life to the fetus would cause more harm to it than denying it life through abortion. Because of the poor quality of life the child would have if born, abortion can be seen as being in the best interest of the child himself or herself (19).
- *Aborting abnormal fetuses benefits society as a whole.* Abortion brings about a substantial saving of societal resources that would otherwise be used for the special care and education of children suffering from serious diseases. These resources can be used for individuals who are able to make return contributions to society (18).

It should be noted that these arguments are in accord with a *utilitarian* approach to ethics (see Chapter 1). The utilitarian looks at consequences of actions in judging their rightness and wrongness, and maintains that the right action to perform is the one having the best consequences for everyone who will be affected by the action, including society as a whole.

Persons who are pro-life and opposed to abortion under any circumstances are likely to try to counter these arguments with the following points:

- With some diseases and disorders, the severity of the symptoms varies from individual to individual. For example, Down's syndrome is a genetically based disorder which involves certain characteristic physical features (such as short stature, flat face, tongue protruding through thick lips) as well as mental impairment. However, the degree of mental impairment can range from severe to slight (20). Even identical twins with cystic fibrosis can differ in how much they show the symptoms of the disease (21). Prenatal diagnosis only indicates whether the child will be affected by a particular disease or disorder; it does not provide information about its severity. One could abort a child who would be only mildly affected by a disease or disorder.

■ Even though a child suffers from a disease or disorder, he can still have a good quality of life. The disease or disorder is not the totality of the person. The child may have distinct abilities—artistic talents, wit, or intellect—that make life enjoyable for him as well as enabling him to contribute to society (22). An example is Blaine Deatherage-Newsome who has spina bifida, is paralyzed from the armpits down, and is confined to a wheel chair; nevertheless, he was also an A student in high school and a national chess champion (23). This is how Blaine describes his life:

> "I was born with spina bifida and hydrocephalus. I hear that when parents have a test and find out that their unborn child has spina bifida, in more than 95 percent of the cases they choose to have an abortion. I also went to an exhibit at the Oregon Museum of Science and Industry several years ago where the exhibit described a child born with spina bifida and hydrocephalus, and . . . asked people to vote on whether the child should live or die. I voted that the child should live, but when I voted, the child was losing by quite a few votes.
>
> When these things happen, I get worried. I wonder if people are saying that they think the world would be a better place without me. I wonder if people just think the lives of people with disabilities are so full of misery and suffering that they think we would be better off dead. It's true that my life has suffering (especially when I'm having one of my eleven surgeries so far), but most of the time I am very happy and I like my life very much. My mom says she can't imagine the world without me, and she is convinced that everyone who has a chance to know me thinks that the world is a far better place because I'm in it" (23).

■ Having a child with a serious disease or disorder does not necessarily cause an unhappy family life. In fact, such a child can enrich the life of the family. As one study group from the Hastings Center noted: "Families with children who are seriously ill or disabled often can find meaning and satisfaction in their lives, despite many obstacles. They are able to derive genuine joy from their children, as do other parents. They discover that their mutual commitment to the child has created an increased closeness among their members, 'involvement,' and personal growth. Siblings, by their own accounts, have become more sensitive and caring adults due to their experiences in helping to care for a seriously ill or disabled family member" (24).

Perhaps the most difficult decisions regarding selective abortion involve prenatal diagnosis of abnormalities which are very likely to be fatal shortly after birth (2), such as anencephaly, in which a baby is born without parts of the brain and skull (25), and Patau Syndrome, a trisomy of chromosome 13 (26). Whether an abortion is performed or not, the baby will die (2). Having an abortion will at least spare the mother the burden of continuing with the pregnancy and giving birth and the trauma of waiting for the newborn to die (2).

On the other hand, there are some physical risks involved with having an abortion. Surgical abortion involves "such risks as pelvic infection, blood clots in the uterus, heavy bleeding, cut or torn cervix, perforation of the uterus wall, and anesthesia-related complications" (27). Medical (medication) abortions using Mifeprex and misoprostol may have side effects of nausea, weakness, fever/chills, vomiting, headache, diarrhea and dizziness (28). More serious complications include the possibility of prolonged heavy bleeding and bacterial infection (29).

There has been controversy about emotional effects of abortion on women (2, 30, 31). For present purposes, a statement in an article on this subject from Planned Parenthood is noteworthy: ". . . most substantive studies in the last 30 years have found abortion to be a relatively benign procedure in terms of emotional effect—except when pre-abortion emotional problems exist or when a wanted pregnancy is terminated, such as after diagnostic genetic testing" (30). The second exception is applicable to our case study regarding abortion in the case of fetuses with cystic fibrosis.

Abortion in the Case of Rape

When a woman voluntarily engages in sexual relations knowing the risks of conceiving a child (and we know that no method of artificial contraception is 100 percent effective), then it might be argued that she gives any child conceived the right to use her body. This simply does not apply, however, in the case of rape, where sex is forced upon a woman against her will. Some who are generally against abortion are still willing to allow it in those rare cases in which conception occurs as the result of rape. Thus, abortion in the case of rape deserves special attention.

It is generally accepted that there can be morally legitimate cases of killing in self-defense. Some argue that a woman who has been raped is simply defending herself against the attack in having an abortion (32). However, those totally opposed to abortion might claim that the self-defense justification for killing is being incorrectly applied here. First of all, they might point out that the rapist, not the fetus, is the aggressor against whom the woman may take protective action. Further, there is a sense in which the fetus too is a victim of the rapist, in that the fetus was conceived in circumstances in which it was not wanted.

No one denies that it is traumatic and very difficult for a woman who is pregnant as a result of rape to carry the fetus to term. Nevertheless, in this situation an opponent of abortion from the Christian religious tradition might appeal to the New Testament parable of the Good Samaritan:

> A man was going down from Jerusalem to Jericho, when he fell into the hands of robbers. They stripped him of his clothes, beat him and went away, leaving him half dead. A priest happened to be going down the same road, and when he saw the man, he passed by on the other side. So too, a Levite, when he came to the place and saw him, passed by on the other side. But a Samaritan, as he traveled, came where the man was; and when he saw him, he took pity on him. He went to him and bandaged his wounds, pouring on oil and wine. Then he put the man on his own donkey, took him to an inn and took care of him. The next day he took out two silver coins, and gave them to the innkeeper. "Look after him," he said, "and when I return, I will reimburse you for any extra expense you may have."
>
> "Which of these three do you think was a neighbor to the man who fell into the hands of robbers?"
>
> The expert in the law replied, "The one who had mercy on him."
>
> Jesus told him, "Go and do likewise." (Luke 10: 30–37)

The point of this story is that the "Good Samaritan went out of his way, at some cost to himself, to help one in need of it" (32). Philosophical ethicists might call this an *act of supererogation:* an act which is morally commendable but which no one can be expected or obliged to perform. Similarly, it might be categorized as an act of supererogation for a woman who has been raped to carry the fetus to term in order to give the child life (32). However, working within a religious framework, a woman might be strongly encouraged to go beyond what is strictly required and refrain from having an abortion.

CHAPTER SUMMARY

Key Terms and Concepts

abortion: the termination of a pregnancy with resulting death of the human fetus.

spontaneous abortion: a miscarriage; the termination of a pregnancy caused by purely natural factors.

induced or procured abortion: the termination of a pregnancy caused by human action.

indirect abortion: one type of induced/procured abortion occurring when the direct, immediate purpose of a procedure is to treat the mother for a threatening pathology, but the death of the fetus is also an inevitable secondary result.

direct abortion: one type of induced/procured abortion occurring when the direct, immediate purpose of the procedure is to destroy the human fetus or to expel it when it is not viable. The term "abortion" as commonly used refers to direct abortion.

selective abortion: abortion of a fetus because it has certain unwanted characteristics, usually abnormalities.

Key Points

- Three different positions have been taken on the moral permissibility of abortion: (a) abortion on demand; that is, the view that abortion is permissible at any time during a pregnancy for any reason whatever; (b) the view that abortion is permissible in a limited number of cases (e.g., rape, incest, fetal abnormality, when the pregnancy threatens the well-being of the mother); and (c) the view that abortion is never permissible.
- Abortion is debated in terms of rights possessed by the mother and by the fetus respectively. In support of abortion, the following claims are made:
  * A woman has a right to a normal sex life, and is entitled to use abortion when artificial contraception fails.
  * A woman has a right to control what happens to her body.
- In opposition to abortion, the following claims about rights are made:
  * When a woman voluntarily engages in sexual relations, she gives any child who may be conceived the right to use her body.
  * The fetus's right to life takes precedence over hardships which may be experienced by the mother due to pregnancy and/or caregiving responsibilities for a child.

- One very common argument against abortion is that it is the killing of an innocent human being. This argument assumes that the embryo/fetus is a human being.
- Exactly when human life begins remains a matter of controversy.
- A utilitarian line of argument to justify aborting abnormal fetuses is that abortion will prevent suffering for both the family and the child and that it will benefit society by saving resources.
- Those opposed to aborting abnormal fetuses make the following points:
  * Families having a child with a serious disease can still have a happy and satisfying family life.
  * A child with a serious disease can still have abilities that enable the child to enjoy a good quality of life.
  * With some diseases, the severity of the symptoms varies from individual to individual, so that one could abort a child who would only be mildly affected.
  * A disease is not the totality of the person; persons suffering from diseases can make positive contributions to society through abilities they possess.
- Surgical and medical (medication) abortions carry certain physical risks; there may also be emotional effects on some women who have abortions.
- Some who are generally against abortion consider it permissible in the case of rape. Abortion in this case is defended on grounds of self-defense. However, there are also people who encourage women who have been raped to make the sacrifice of carrying the pregnancy to term in order to give the child the gift of life.

FOR FURTHER DISCUSSION

1. Abortion is a very controversial issue. This chapter has set out the arguments both for and against the moral permissibility of abortion in various cases. Looking at these arguments, which of the following positions do you personally adopt on the abortion issue?

   - abortion on demand (that is, abortion is permissible at any time during a pregnancy for any reason);
   - abortion is permissible only in certain cases (specify which ones);
   - abortion is never permissible.

   What reasons can you give to defend the position you take?

2. Divide the class into groups representing the three positions listed in (1) earlier. Then have a formal debate about the positions.
3. This chapter has set out the reasons for citing various times during embryonic and fetal development as the beginning of human life. Looking at the evidence, at what time do you personally think that human life begins? What reasons are persuasive to you?

References

1. Benedict M. Ashley, O.P. and Kevin D. O'Rourke, O.P., *Health Care Ethics: A Theological Analysis*, 4th ed. (Washington, DC: Georgetown University Press, 1997).
2. Christopher Kaczor, *The Ethics of Abortion Women's Rights, Human Life, and the Questions of Justice*, 2nd ed. (New York: Routledge, 2015).
3. Judith Jarvis Thompson, "A Defense of Abortion," *Philosophy and Public Affairs* 1/1 (Fall 1971): 47–66.
4. Mary Anne Warren, "On the Moral and Legal Status of Abortion," *Monist* 57/1 (January 1973): 43–61.
5. *Roev. Wade* 410 United States Reports 113; decided January 22, 1973.
6. Daniel Callahan, "How Technology Is Reframing the Abortion Debate," *Hastings Center Report* (February 1986): 34.
7. John T. Noonan, Jr., "An Almost Absolute Value in History," in John T. Noonan, Jr. (ed.), *The Morality of Abortion: Legal and Historical Perspectives* (Cambridge, MA: Harvard, 1970).
8. Ronald Munson, *Intervention and Reflection Basic Issues in Medical Ethics*, 8th ed. (Belmont, CA: Thomson Wadsworth, 2008).
9. Robert P. George and Christopher Tollefsen, *Embryo A Defense of Human Life* (New York: Doubleday, 2008).
10. Rem B. Edwards and Glenn C. Graber, "Concepts of Death," in Rem B. Edwards and Glenn C. Graber (eds.), *Bioethics* (San Diego: Harcourt Brace Jovanovich, 1988).
11. Andre E. Hellegers, "Fetal Development," *Theological Studies* 31/1 (March 1970): 3–9.
12. Ronald M. Green, *The Human Embryo Research Debates* (New York: Oxford University Press, 2001).
13. Marc Ramsey, "Twinning and Fusion as Arguments against the Moral Standing of the Early Human Embryo," *Utilitas* 23/2 (June 2011): 183–205.

14. Patrick Lee and Robert P. George, "The First Fourteen Days of Human Life," *The New Atlantis* (Summer 2006): 61–67.15.

15. Robert P. George and Alfonso Gomez-Lobo, "The Moral Status of the Human Embryo," *Perspectives in Biology and Medicine* 48 (2005): 201–10.

16. Kevin T. Fitzgerald, "Human Embryonic Stem Cell Research: Ethics in the Face of Uncertainty," in Brent Walters and Ronald Cole-Turner (eds.), *God and the Embryo Religious Voices on Stem Cells and Cloning* (Washington, DC: Georgetown University Press, 2003), 131–40.

17. Tom L. Beauchamp and LeRoy Walters, *Contemporary Issues in Bioethics*, 6th ed. (Belmont, CA: Thomson Wadsworth, 2003).

18. Leon R. Kass, "Implications of Prenatal Diagnosis for the Human Right to Life," in Bruce Hilton, Daniel Callahan, Maureen Harris, Peter Condliffe, and Burton Berkeley (eds.), *Ethical Issues in Human Genetics: Genetic Counseling and the Use of Genetic Knowledge* (New York: Plenum, 1973)

19. Edmund N. Santurri, "Prenatal Diagnosis: Some Moral Considerations," in Edward D. Schneider (ed.), *Questions about the Beginning of Life* (Minneapolis: Augsburg, 1985).

20. Ricki Lewis, *Human Genetics*, 5th ed. (New York: McGraw-Hill, 2003).

21. Panel on cystic fibrosis, College Course 25, "Ethical, Legal, and Social Implications of the Human Genome Project," Dartmouth College, July 2, 1997.

22. Adrienne Asch, College Course 25, *Ethical, Legal and Social Implications of the Human Genome Project* (Dartmouth College, Hanover, NH, July 10, 1997).

23. Ricki Lewis, *Human Genetics Concepts and Applications*, 2nd ed. (Dubuque, IA: Wm. C. Brown, 1997).

24. Arthur Caplan and Cynthia B. Cohen (eds.), "Imperiled Newborns," Hastings Center Project Report, *Hastings Center Report* 17/6 (December 1987): 5–31.

25. Centers for Disease Control and Prevention, *Facts about Anencephaly*. http://www.cdc.gov.ncbddd/birthdefects/anencephaly.html Accessed March 2016.

26. Medscape, *Patau Syndrome*. http://emedicine.medscape.com/article/947706-overview. Accessed March 2016.

27. David Boonin, *A Defense of Abortion* (New York: Cambridge University Press, 2003).

28. FDA, *Medication Guide: Mifeprex*. http://www.fda.gov/downloads/Drugs/DrugSafety/ucmo88643.pdf. Accessed March 2016.

29. FDA, *Mifeprex Prescribing Information* http://www.accessdata.fda.gov /drugsatfda_docs/label/2005/020687s013lbl.pdf Accessed March 2016.
30. Planned Parenthood, *The Emotional Effects of Induced Abortion.* https:// www.plannedparenthood.org/files/8413/9611/5708/Abortion_ Emotional_Effects.pdf Accessed March 2016.
31. Thomas W. Strahan (ed.), *Detrimental Effects of Abortion: An Annotated Bibliography with Commentary*, 3rd ed. (Springfield, IL: Acorn Books, 2001).
32. Jane English, "Abortion and the Concept of a Person," *Canadian Journal of Philosophy* 5/2 (October 1975): 233–43.

Chapter 4

Assisted Reproductive Technologies

The way we can go about having children has been dramatically changed by the development of assisted reproductive technologies (ART). Artificial insemination, in vitro fertilization, donor eggs, donor sperm, embryo freezing, egg banking, and surrogate motherhood are all technologies available to assist people in having a much wanted child (1). First and foremost, these technologies are intended to assist married couples overcome problems of infertility. However, the use of these technologies has been extended to enable single persons and members of the LGBT community to have children (1).

When one sees the happiness of people who have a child when they thought they could never have one at all, it seems one can only express gratitude for the technologies that make this possible. Nevertheless, some have voiced concerns about these technologies from an ethical point of view.

In this chapter, you will learn about:

- Ethical issues that have been raised about such assisted reproductive technologies as artificial insemination by donor, in vitro fertilization, and surrogacy;
- How concerns about assisted reproductive technologies interface with ethical theories.

Case Study

Ellen Peterson has just completed her educational training as a clinical laboratory technologist. One of her professors has recommended her for a job at a nearby university fertility clinic, and she has been called to come for a job interview.

As part of the interview process, Ellen meets with the clinic's director. She finds the director tremendously enthusiastic about the kind of work being done at the clinic to help infertile couples realize their dream of having a child. The director tells her the story of one couple who had recently used the clinic's services.

"The couple had married in their late twenties, after completing graduate school," he stated. "After trying unsuccessfully to become pregnant for 2 years, the wife decided to see a doctor who is a fertility specialist for a work-up. No problems were detected. She then convinced her husband to see the doctor. Testing indicated that her husband is infertile. He is producing almost no sperm. However, the doctor told them not to lose hope in their dream of having a family, and referred them to our fertility clinic to explore the technologies currently available to assist infertile couples in having children. The couple came to our clinic and decided to use the procedure of artificial insemination by donor (AID). A pregnancy was achieved using AID. Just this morning the couple visited our clinic to show off their new baby daughter and to thank our staff for their help!"

Ellen can appreciate the joy the clinic's work has brought to this couple by enabling them to have a much wanted child. At the same time, Ellen herself comes from a religious background that considers the use of donor sperm equivalent to an act of adultery. Before she accepts a position at this clinic, she wants some time to reflect on the ethics of the procedures the clinic is performing.

■ ■ ■

Artificial Insemination by Donor

Artificial insemination (AI) is a fertilization procedure in which a fine catheter (tube) is used to deposit sperm into a woman's cervix (intracervical insemination—ICI) or into her uterus (intrauterine insemination—IUI). The sperm may come either from the woman's husband (AIH) or from a donor (AID) (2, 3).

Artificial insemination by husband (AIH) may be used in the case of problems with suboptimal semen quality, premature ejaculation, impotence, and retrograde ejaculation inside the urinary bladder after prostate surgery (4, 5). AIH may also be used when the male partner has undergone a vasectomy but would subsequently like to have a child (5). AIH can also be used with sperm obtained and frozen before men undergo chemotherapy or radiation treatments for cancer (4, 5). AIH may also be used to bypass cervical problems in women, such as a narrowed cervix or absent, abnormally thick or acidic cervical mucus (4).

Artificial insemination by donor (AID) may be sought by a married couple "if the male partner suffers from severe sperm problems (extremely low count, no motile sperm, no sperm with normal morphology, sperm without the ability to penetrate the egg or the complete absence of sperm)" (6). Or again, a couple may seek AID for genetic reasons; for example, when the husband is the carrier of a dominant gene for a genetic disorder or when both husband and wife are carriers of a recessive gene for a genetic disorder (6, 7). Thus, this procedure has sometimes been referred to as *therapeutic donor insemination (TDI)* (6).

Ethically, we will focus on artificial insemination by donor (AID).

In the case study Ellen Peterson alludes to one ethical concern that has been expressed about AID in the case of a heterosexual married couple: it involves going outside the bond of the marriage to have a child. Some see it as part of the very meaning of marriage that the spouses pledge to have children only through each other (8). Anecdotal evidence indicates that feelings of infidelity can accompany the use of AID by married couples:

> A couple who had been treated for male infertility for three years had just finished their second and last IVF cycle in which they did not get fertilization. . . . They made an appointment with the psychologist to discuss donor insemination. The husband stated that he was ready to move on to DI [donor insemination]. . . . His wife was far more hesitant, telling the psychologist timidly, "I've never told anyone this, but my husband is the only man I have ever had sex with. I'm afraid that having another man's sperm inside me would make me feel like I was sleeping with someone else."

Men similarly may express feelings of hesitancy about DI due to fears that if their wife conceives, they will feel as if she is carrying another man's child. (7)

The same ethical concern about breaking the marital covenant would apply to any technology involving the use of donor sperm or donor ova by a heterosexual married couple.

Another ethical issue pertains to the sperm donor himself. Someone can donate blood, and then just walk away. But donating sperm seems different. It has more significant consequences: a new human life is produced through artificial insemination. Thus the question has been raised of whether, from an ethical point of view, a sperm donor has any responsibilities to the child produced using his sperm, and if so, how this impacts the individuals who are raising his biological child (9).

One approach to ethics—utilitarianism—makes judgments of rightness and wrongness based on the consequences of a course of action for everyone affected (see Chapter 1). On the one hand, AID is seen as having benefits (good consequences) for a couple in comparison with adoption. Specifically, both the husband and wife can be involved in the pregnancy from conception onward, sharing the experience of delivery and the early days of the baby's life. The desire on the part of the mother to carry a child is satisfied as it cannot be in adoption. Further, the husband and wife can exercise control over the child's prenatal care and need not worry that something in the prenatal environment may cause problems later in the child's life. Moreover, there is a greater chance that the child's physical appearance will at least match that of the mother and, if there are several children, they are more likely to resemble one another. There also need be no subconscious fear of the sudden appearance of the natural mother, as there may be in adoption. Finally, AID affords privacy to a couple while adoption is a public statement about their infertility (7, 10, 11).

On the other hand, there can be negative psychological consequences for a couple using AID. A Canadian study of 120 couples using AID indicated that use of this procedure "generates intense and troublesome feelings both within and between spouses" (7). The researchers found that "common reactions for men are loss of self-esteem, emotional withdrawal, and temporary impotence" (7). For their part, women experience "anger, guilt, and a wish to make reparations" (7).

Moreover, AID carries the negative consequence of a loss of genetic continuity. While most children "have some qualities of each parent that are recognizable," couples considering the use of AID "must face their feelings of sadness about not being able to see some of the father's traits reflected in their children" (7). Further, couples who have a strong sense of family roots may feel that donor insemination is severing their ancestral ties and that they may disappoint their families by choosing AID. They may also worry that, if their family learns about their use of AID, the grandchild will not be loved or accepted in the same way a biological child would be (7).

AID may also have some negative consequences for the child. If the sperm donor is anonymous, lack of knowledge of the child's paternal heritage may prove harmful if the child should need a reliable family medical history (12). Further, with the practice of anonymous donation comes the possibility of sibling marriages (12).

There can similarly be negative ramifications for the sperm donor and those with whom he is in relationship. A sperm donor must face the fact that "he will have offspring whom he will not know" (7). Further, "if the donor has children of his own, they will have half-siblings whom they do not know," and the donor "must think about whether he would tell his children about their unknown genetic siblings" (7). A sperm donor must also "consider whether he will tell his spouse (or future spouse) and how his spouse might react to the information" (7).

In sum, a utilitarian in ethics would weigh both the positive and negative consequences for the whole range of affected persons in making a judgment about the rightness or wrongness of AID (see Chapter 1).

It is noteworthy that AID has been used as part of a eugenic program to produce superior human beings. One such program was the Repository for Germinal Choice in San Marcos, California, whose donors of germinal material consisted of Nobel Laureates in science and other high achievers. The recipients were young women selected for their superior health and intellect, under 35 years of age, with sterile husbands who agreed to the use of AID. The aim of the project was to increase the number of offspring of the most creative scientists of our time (13). In a similar vein, the Fairfax Cryobank in Fairfax, Virginia, has a special category of sperm donors called "Fairfax Graduate," consisting of donors who "are in the process of earning or have completed a post college graduate degree" (14). These individuals include "masters level degrees, medical, dental, chiropractic, law (Juris doctorate), veterinary, optometry, pharmacy, and Ph.D. students and graduates" (14).

Our case study and discussion of it have focused on the use of AID by heterosexual married couples. However, some single women and lesbian couples have used AID in order to bear a child (15). In conjunction with surrogacy, AID can also be used by single men or gay men to have a child.

Case Study

Chuck Forbes works as a physician assistant at a fertility clinic which is part of a university hospital and medical school. He sometimes conducts the initial interview with couples coming to the clinic for the first time.

Today Chuck has an interview with Rita and John Linden. Rita and John are now in their mid-thirties. When they got married after college they decided to postpone having children until they both got established in their careers and had achieved some degree of financial security. Four years ago they decided they were ready to start a family, but their efforts to conceive a child never resulted in a pregnancy. It was discovered that Rita had blocked fallopian tubes which prevented ova from reaching her uterus. She underwent surgical repair of her oviducts, but still could not conceive. The Lindens' physician has suggested they go to the fertility clinic to investigate in vitro fertilization (IVF).

Rita and John have heard concerns expressed by friends at their church about the fate of embryos in the IVF process. They tell Chuck Forbes that they want to be fully informed about the IVF procedure before they make a decision to go this route to try to have a child.

■ ■ ■

In Vitro Fertilization

In vitro fertilization (IVF) involves stimulating multiple ova to develop, retrieving them from the woman, fertilizing them in the laboratory with sperm, and transferring resulting embryos to a woman's body to attempt to achieve a pregnancy (16). The ova and sperm used in the IVF process can either come from a married couple, or one or both can be donated (17, 18). Intracytoplasmic sperm injection (ICSI) may be used in conjunction with IVF. In this procedure sperm are directly injected into the eggs to achieve fertilization (16). Embryos not immediately transferred to a woman are typically frozen for later use (12).

Multifetal pregnancies (twins, triplets, or more) can result if too many embryos are transferred to a woman at a given time. Thus the number of embryos transferred is determined by the quality of the embryos and by weighing the risks for a multifetal pregnancy against the risk of failing to conceive since, as female age increases, the implantation rate of embryos tends to decline (16). If they occur, multifetal pregnancies, especially high-order multiples, pose serious health risks for both the mother and the developing fetuses (19). Selective reduction may be undertaken in such cases, that is, the life of one or more of the fetuses will be terminated (19). One's judgment about the ethical permissibility of selective reduction is dependent on one's views about the human and moral status of the fetus (see Chapter 3).

One book for people thinking about using IVF has a section entitled "IVF Requires a Heavy Emotional, Physical, and Financial Investment" and another section entitled "IVF is an Emotional, Physical, and Financial Roller-Coaster Ride" (19). Undergoing IVF is stressful in a number of respects. Couples have to deal with the feelings of shame, guilty, anxiety, depression, and anger that have resulted with their long-standing battle with infertility. They may have to travel to a different and unfamiliar geographical location to access the IVF treatment, and interact with strange and sometimes impersonal clinical staff. The drugs that must be taken by the woman may trigger unpredictable emotions. IVF is very expensive, and may not be covered by insurance. Finally, there is the waiting to see if the procedure will work, with the very real possibility of failure (19).

Ethically, the principle of nonmaleficence directs us to avoid taking actions that bring harm to others (see Chapter 1). Thus, there is concern whether IVF poses physical risks to the children conceived through this technology.

For example, in 2012 researchers reported to a conference of the American Academy of Pediatrics that "IVF may significantly increase birth defect risk, especially in the heart, eyes, reproductive organs and urinary systems" (20). Specifically, among the infants in the study "9% . . . born after IVF had birth defects compared to 6.6% of babies who were conceived naturally" (20). The possibility was considered that "the higher rate of abnormalities with IVF is due in part to whatever was contributing to infertility in the first place" (20). However, the researchers concluded that "the fact that an increase [in birth defects] was not seen among babies conceived using artificial insemination or ovulation induction suggest that the process of IVF itself . . . is the primary culprit" (20).

Another study found that "the increased risk of birth defects associated with IVF was no longer significant after adjustment for parental factors" although "the risk of birth defects associated with ICSI remained increased after multivariate adjustment" (21). At the same time, "a recent meta-analysis looking at ICSI vs. IVF" concluded that "there is no additional risk connected to ICSI" (22). In sum, further study is needed before a definitive judgment can be made on IVF and risks for birth defects.

In the case study, Rita and John Linden express concern about the fate of the embryos created in the IVF process. Embryonic loss does occur with IVF. It is known that not all the embryos transferred to a woman will implant to achieve a viable pregnancy (16). Further, frozen embryos can become "spare" if a couple does not want to use them for further attempts to achieve a pregnancy. A couple may achieve the number of children they desire and not want more. Or repeated attempts at embryo transfer may not work to achieve a pregnancy and the couple becomes discouraged and stops trying. Or there may simply be too many frozen embryos to reasonably transfer all of them back to the biological mother to have additional children. It has been estimated that there are now about 400,000–600,000 human embryos existing in a frozen state, with only about 10,000 a year being thawed to be given life in a family (23). Thus the disposition of excess frozen embryos is a major issue accompanying the practice of in vitro fertilization.

One option is for a couple to decide that their spare frozen embryos should simply be disposed of by the reproductive clinic storing them (24). The ethical permissibility of this option is dependent on one's views about the human and moral status of the early state embryo (see Chapter 3).

Another option is for the couple to donate their spare frozen embryos for scientific research, notably, for stem cell research. The ethics of this option will be discussed at length in Chapter 18. However, it can be noted that this option also involves loss of life for the embryos.

Yet another option is long-term storage of spare frozen embryos until they naturally "die," that is, when they reach a state when they can no longer be thawed and be viable to achieve a pregnancy. However, one practical problem with this option is when a frozen embryo in fact "dies." The biological parents of frozen embryos have come back to fertility clinics "after 10–12 years and the embryos have been thawed successfully and created healthy babies" (24). In 2013 a birth was reported from an embryo which had been frozen for 19 years (23). Indeed, it is being reported by fertility clinics that "with the rapid advances in reproductive medicine, cryopreserved or frozen embryos can potentially remain viable for an indefinite period of time" (25). However, in the United Kingdom it is government policy that all embryos in frozen storage for more than 5 years be destroyed (24). No such laws or policies have yet been established in the United States but it is not inconceivable that such policies could be instituted here if a very large number of spare frozen embryos are being kept in storage for a long period of time.

A final option is for a couple to donate their spare frozen embryos for adoption by other couples. Agencies have been established precisely for this purpose (26, 27).

Some are also concerned that technological methods of reproduction, such as IVF, which separate the conception of a child from an interpersonal act of sexual intercourse and make it into a purely laboratory procedure, will create a mentality of viewing children as "commodities to be manufactured." As stated by one couple who tried such technological methods:

> Paul Lauritzen, speaking for himself and his wife, sums up the experience of their efforts to generate children through technological processes by saying: "The process of reproduction in a clinical environment (causes) a way of thinking of ourselves and our world in terms that are incompatible with intimacy . . . once procreation is separated from sexual intercourse, it is difficult not to treat the process of procreation as the *production of an object to which one has the right as a producer.*" (28; italics added)

A mentality of treating our children as "objects" would violate Kantian ethics (see Chapter 1).

There is also concern that the use of donor sperm or ova with IVF and other reproductive technologies can lead to disruption and confusion of parent-child and family relationships. Scenarios such as the following are not far-fetched. Suppose that Sally, a woman in her mid-forties who is divorced, decides to remarry and that she and her new husband (who is a childless widower) want to start a family. Sally is now infertile, and consultation with an IVF clinic indicates that she is not a suitable candidate for that procedure. However, the clinic does tell the couple that the husband's sperm could be used to fertilize a donor egg, and that the embryo could be implanted in a surrogate mother who would carry the child to term for them. Sally has a daughter in her twenties from her previous marriage, and the daughter offers to donate the ovum to be used in the IVF procedure so that the child will be genetically related to Sally. Thus Sally will be in the unusual position of being both mother (in terms of social relationships) and grandmother (biologically) to the child, and Sally's daughter will be both the child's mother (biologically) and its sister (in terms of social relationships) (29).

In the future, a child could have three sets of parents. The child could be conceived in vitro from ova and sperm coming from a man and woman who may be either living or dead (frozen sperm or ova). A surrogate mother could carry the child to term, and then surrender the child to yet another couple to raise him or her. In other words, reproductive technologies have the potential to separate *biological* parenting from *gestational* parenting from *social* parenting (30). What will this kind of separation do to a child psychologically? And to the child's sense of personal identity?

Case Study

Jerry Zellner has worked in the laboratory of the Wentworth Fertility Clinic for the past five years. The clinic's programs include gestatational surrogacy services. Recently the clinic's director asked him to serve on a special committee to deal with a problem situation.

At the first committee meeting, Jerry learns about the situation that brought about the formation of the committee. A surrogate recently gave birth to twins. The couple who contracted with the surrogate is refusing to take two babies. They claim they legally agreed to have only one child, and they have already picked out the one they want. The surrogate is married with two sons of her own, and decided to work as a surrogate mother to earn some extra money for her own family. Financially, she can't possibly assume care of yet another child.

The committee must make recommendations concerning the fate of the two babies. If the contracting couple succeeds in their claim to assume care of only one of the babies, who should decide which one they get? Does the surrogate have any responsibilities for the second child since she carried it and brought it to birth? Should arrangements be made to put the second child up for adoption?

Apart from these immediate concerns, one committee member suggests that the clinic undertake a comprehensive study of its surrogacy services to prevent problems for the clinic in the future. Jerry concurs with this suggestion, commenting that the study should address the ethical dimensions of surrogacy as well as clinical and legal issues. He has come to wonder if we as a society need to be more selective in our use of reproductive technologies.

■ ■ ■

Surrogacy

Surrogacy takes several forms. In traditional surrogacy, a woman is artificially inseminated with the commissioning male's sperm and carries the pregnancy with a pledge to give the child to the contracting couple or male once it is born. The surrogate is genetically related to the child since she has contributed the egg (31). More prevalent today is gestational surrogacy, in which ova and sperm are fertilized in vitro and then developing embryos are transferred to the surrogate who carries the pregnancy with the intent of giving the child to those who created the embryo once the child is born. In this case, the surrogate is not genetically related to the child (31). Medical indications for resort to a gestational surrogate include an absent uterus, recurrent miscarriage, or repeated failure of IVF (31). A woman may be hired through an agency to serve as a gestational surrogate for monetary compensation (commercial surrogacy), or a relative or friend may offer to serve as a gestational surrogate without monetary compensation (altruistic surrogacy) (32). The case study with the Wentworth Fertility Clinic involves commercial gestational surrogacy.

Gestational surrogacy can be attractive to a couple with infertility problems because it is a quicker and less cumbersome procedure than legal adoption (32). Further, it gives the couple a child who is related to them genetically (31).

At the same time, there are potential complications in using gestational surrogacy. One issue is the degree to which the surrogate mother is autonomous and to what extent the genetic parents may impose their wishes and demands on her style of living, habits and health (33). For example, may the genetic parents force the surrogate mother to undergo prenatal diagnosis? And, depending on the results, can the surrogate mother be forced to terminate the pregnancy? (33) Or suppose that the child is born handicapped or mentally challenged and the genetic parents do not wish to accept it. What will be the fate of the child? (34) Or again, suppose that the genetic parents divorce or unexpectedly die before the birth of the child? What will happen to the child? (34) As illustrated in the case study, a surrogate mother may not be able or willing to accept a child abandoned by its genetic parents.

Surrogacy is clearly an issue of particular concern to women. Feminists have been split in their assessment of surrogacy. Some have defended the practice on the grounds that women should be allowed to control their own bodies, with surrogacy being one of their reproductive choices (33, 35). Other feminists have opposed surrogacy. It is seen as an affront to the dignity of women: "When a woman provides womb service, the feminist issue surfaces. Women object to being baby factories or sex objects because it offends their human dignity" (35). Indeed, surrogate motherhood has been compared to prostitution (3334,–35).

The monetary payment that accompanies commercial surrogacy carries the danger of exploiting women who are poor. Such monetary compensation can put pressure on poor women to use their bodies to support themselves and their families (36). It is feared that "it is always going to be poor women who have the babies and rich women who get them" (35).

These concerns about commercial surrogacy are illustrated by the "reproductive tourism" that has developed in India (37). Americans have gone to India to hire gestational surrogates because "surrogacy costs about $12,000 in India, including all medical expenses and the surrogate's fee" while in the United States "the same procedure can cost up to $70,000" (37). An article in *Marie*

Claire magazine describes the situation of Indian women attracted to serve as gestational surrogates:

> Vohra has no job but helps her husband in his scrap-metal business, for which they earn 50 to 60 rupees ($1.20 to $1.45) a day. If her pregnancy is successful, the $5,500 she receives will, as she puts it, "give my children a future."
>
> Growing up, Vohra worked in the wheat fields; she had little education. After her parents married her off at 16, she moved with her husband into a one-room mud house that erodes every year during the monsoon season. She plans to divide her surrogacy windfall three ways: buying a brick house, investing in her husband's business, and paying for her children's education. "My daughter wants to be a teacher," she says. "I'll do anything to give her that opportunity." (37)

Or again, the article tells the story of Rubina Mondal whose 8-year-old son has a hole in his heart and who decided to work as a surrogate in order to cover his medical expenses (37).

In 2015 the Indian Council of Medical Research "instructed the country's fertility clinics to stop providing surrogacy services for clients from abroad" (38). This directive is "part of a government effort to impose tighter limits on a growing industry that critics say exploits poor, local women" (38).

Thus surrogate motherhood interfaces with Kant's ethics (see Chapter 1). Does surrogacy—especially commercial surrogacy—simply "use" women to produce children for others? Concomitantly, does surrogacy turn children into "commodities" to be produced? Indeed, it has been argued that "the widespread acceptance of commercial surrogacy would psychologically threaten all children" (39). This is because "it would change the way children are valued by people (parents and surrogate brokers)—from being loved by their parents and respected by others, to being sometimes used as objects of commercial profit-making" (39).

CHAPTER SUMMARY

Key Terms and Concepts

assisted reproductive technologies (ART): medical technologies aimed at helping people have children.

artificial insemination (AI): a fertilization procedure in which a fine catheter (tube) is used to deposit sperm into a woman's cervix (intracervical insemination—**ICI**) or into her uterus (intrauterine insemination—**IUI**). The sperm may come either from the woman's husband **(AIH)** or from a donor **(AID)**.

in vitro fertilization (IVF): a procedure that involves stimulating multiple ova to develop, retrieving them from the woman, fertilizing them in the laboratory with sperm, and transferring resulting embryos to a woman's body to attempt to achieve a pregnancy.

Intracytoplasmic sperm injection (ICSI): a procedure which may be used in conjunction with IVF in which sperm are directly injected into eggs to achieve fertilization.

surrogacy/surrogate motherhood: a reproductive arrangement in which a woman carries a pregnancy with the intent of giving the child, once it is born, to another with whom she has contracted. The pregnancy may be achieved either through artificial insemination with the contracting man's sperm, or by implantation of embryos after in vitro fertilization **(gestational surrogacy)**.

Key Points

- Assisted reproductive technologies have the benefit of enabling people to have a child when they thought they could never have one at all because of problems with infertility. At the same time, ethical concerns have been expressed by some about these technologies.

- While artificial insemination by donor has advantages over adoption, it can also have negative repercussions for the couple using it, the child conceived through this procedure, and the sperm donor himself.

- The use of donor gametes (sperm or ova) by a married couple means going outside their marriage to have a child, and raises the question of breaking their marital covenant to each other.

- In vitro fertilization involves some loss of embryos because not all the embryos transferred to a woman will implant to achieve a pregnancy. There may be additional loss of fetuses because of selective reduction in the case of multifetal pregnancies.

- The disposition of the large number of spare frozen embryos which have resulted from the IVF procedure poses ethical problems. Methods of disposition may involve additional loss and destruction of embryos.

- Whether the procedure of IVF (and ICSI) increases the rate of birth defects is under study.

- There is concern that in vitro fertilization (and other reproductive technologies) will create a mentality of viewing children as commodities as well as lead to disruption and confusion of the parent–child relationship.

- A major concern about the practice of surrogate motherhood is its implications for the treatment and exploitation of women.
- Surrogacy may also have harmful effects on the children involved in this relationship. In some cases, they may be abandoned by the contracting couple. These children may also be regarded as commodities for commercial profit-making.

FOR FURTHER DISCUSSION

1. Michael and Patricia have been married for five years. Both are attorneys, and they now feel that they are sufficiently established in their careers to start a family. Patricia loves music and plays in the community symphony orchestra. While Michael shares her love of music, he doesn't have any musical talent himself and he realizes this. Patricia would really like her children to have musical ability so that their lives could be enriched in this way. Patricia reads about the "Fairfax Graduate" sperm donor program at the Fairfax Cryobank in Virginia (14). She approaches Michael about using this program to obtain sperm donated by a man who generally looks like Michael but who has a doctoral degree in music. Initially, Michael is hurt that Patricia doesn't regard him as good enough to father her children. However, out of love for Patricia and because he himself would like their children to have musical ability, Michael finally agrees to this plan.

    From an ethical point of view, is this a permissible course of action to take?

2. Ginny and Tony, both in their mid-thirties, have started a program of in vitro fertilization. The first two cycles of embryo transfer fail to achieve a pregnancy. Then Ginny unexpectedly becomes pregnant naturally, something the doctors didn't think could happen. In fact, Ginny is carrying twins. Ginny and Tony still have 12 frozen embryos, and they must now decide what to do with them. They must decide among the following options:

    - *Keep the embryos frozen to use in the future to try to have additional children.*
    - *Have the reproductive clinic dispose of the frozen embryos.*
    - *Donate the embryos for scientific research.*
    - *Keep the embryos frozen indefinitely in the hope that they will simply "die."*
    - *Donate the frozen embryos to an agency which will arrange for other couples to adopt them.*

Are there any options which you would rule out as ethically impermissible? And why? From an ethical point of view, which option do you think is the best one for Ginny and Tony to pursue? And why?

3. In the third case study in this chapter, a special committee at the Wentworth Fertility Clinic must deal with a situation in which a surrogate mother has unexpectedly given birth to twins and the contracting couple is unwilling to accept two children. From an ethical point of view, what duties and responsibilities apply to this situation? What recommendations should the committee make regarding the fate of the two babies?

4. The proposal has been put forward that women in a persistent/permanent vegetative state—PVS—(see Chapter 10) might be used as gestational surrogates. There is evidence that this is practically possible:

> . . . in 1996 there was a report of a case of a woman 10 years in PVS (following a car accident), who was raped by a male nurse in the institution where she was hospitalized. She conceived and carried the pregnancy to term, to the delight of the maternal grandparents, whereas the mother remained in PVS for one more year. (33)

Indeed, it has been proposed that "an additional sentence could be appended to the organ donation card, to be signed by women (preferably of reproductive age), willing to serve as gestational surrogates in case an accident renders them to PVS" (33).

> From an ethical point of view, do you think that this is a permissible course of action to pursue? If you are a woman, would you sign a card indicating your willingness to have your body used for gestational surrogacy should you enter a persistent/permanent vegetative state?

References

1. Genetics & IVF Institute, Fairfax, VA http://www.givf.com Accessed April 2016.
2. MedicineNet.com, *MedTerms Medical Dictionary*. http://www.medterms.com. Accessed April 2016.
3. DocShop.com, *Artificial Insemination*. http://www.docshop.com/education/fertility/treatments/ artificial-insemination. Accessed April 2016.

4. Main Line Fertility, *Artificial Insemination: Husband's Sperm (AIH)*. http://www.mainlinefertility.com/artificial-insemination/husbands-sperm. Accessed April 2016.

5. Eugin Clinic, *Artificial Insemination with Partner's Sperm*. https://www.eugin .co.uk/fertility-treatments/artificial-insemination/iac. Accessed April 2016.

6. Infertility, Gynecology, & Obstetrics (IGO) Medical Group of San Diego, *Therapeutic Anonymous Donor Insemination*. http://www.igomed.com/page/infertility. Accessed April 2016

7. Susan Lewis Cooper and Ellen Sarasohn Glazer, *Choosing Assisted Reproduction Social, Emotional & Ethical Considerations* (Indianapolis, IN: Perspectives Press, 1998).

8. Pope Pius XII, "Christian Norms of Morality," in Kevin D. O'Rourke, OP & Philip Boyle, OP, *Medical Ethics: Sources of Catholic Teachings* (St. Louis: Catholic Health Association, 1989).

9. Ronald Munson, "Artificial Insemination and Donor Responsibility," in Ronald Munson (ed.), *Intervention and Reflection Basic Issues in Medical Ethics,* 4th ed. (Belmont, CA: Wadsworth, 1992).

10. Edward D. Schneider, "Artificial Insemination," in Edward D. Schneider (ed.), *Questions About the Beginning of Life* (Minneapolis: Augsburg, 1985).

11. International Federation of Fertility Societies, "International Consensus on Assisted Procreation," *Artificial Insemination With Donor Sperm*. Accessed 2002. http://www.mnet.fr/iffs/a_artbis.htm.

12. Ronald Munson, "Reproductive Control," in Ronald Munson (ed.), *Intervention and Reflection Basic Issues in Medical Ethics,* 8th ed. (Belmont, CA: Thomson Wadsworth, 2008).

13. D. Gareth Jones, *Brave New People* (Grand Rapids, MI: Eerdmans, 1985).

14. Fairfax Cryobank, *About our Donors*. https://www.fairfaxcryobank. com/us/about-our-donors#Categories. Accessed April 2016.

15. Fairfax Cyrobank, *LGBT Families*. https://fairfaxcryobank. com/us/lgbt-families. Accessed April 2016.

16. Advanced Fertility Center of Chicago, In Vitro Fertilization (IVF). http://www.advancedfertility.com. Accessed April 2106.

17. Human Fertilisation & Embryology Authority, *Using Donated Sperm, Eggs, or Embryos in Your Treatment*. http://www.hfea.gov.uk/76.html. Accessed April 2016.

18. Eugin Clinic, *"IVF With Donor Eggs and Donor Sperm."* https://www.eugin.co.uk/fertility-treatments/ivf/donor-eggs-donor-sperm. Accessed April 2016.

19. Geoffrey Sher, Virginia Marriage Davis, and Jean Stoess, *In Vitro Fertilization The A.R.T. of Making Babies* (New York: Skyhorse Publishing, 2013).

20. Alexandra Sifferlin, "*IVF Linked to More Birth Defects*" (October 22, 2012). http://healthland.time.com/2012/10/22/ivf-linked-to-more-birth-defects. Accessed April 2016.

21. Michael J. Davies, Vivienne M. Moore, Kristyn J. Wilson, Phillipa Van Essen, Kevin Priest, Heather Scott, Eric A. Haan, and Annabelle Chan, "Reproductive technologies and the risk of birth defects," *New England Journal of Medicine* 366/19 (May 10, 2012): 1803–13.

22. Anja Pinborg, Anne Loft, Anna-Karina Aaris Henningsen, and Soren Ziebe, "Does Assisted Reproductive Treatment Increase the Risk of Birth Defects in the Offspring?" *Acta Obstetricia et Gynecologica Scandinavica* 91 (2012): 1245–46.

23. Lisa M. Krieger, "Long-frozen Embryo Brings Joy to Adoptive Parents," *San Jose Mercury News.* September 4, 2013. http://www.mercurynews.com/ci_24018720/long-frozen-embryo-brings-joy-adoptive-parents. Accessed April 2016.

24. Pacific Fertility Clinic, *Sperm, Egg, and Embryo Freezing.* http://www.pacificfertilitycenter.com/treatment-care/sperm-egg-and-embryo-freezing. Accessed April 2016.

25. Fairfax Cryobank, *Embryo Storage.* http://www. fairfaxcryobank.com/emstorage.shtml. Accessed April 2016.

26. Embryo Adoption Awareness Center. http://www. embryoadoption.org. Accessed April 2016.

27. Nightlight Christian Adoptions, Snowflakes Embryo Adoption Services. http://www.nightlight.org/snowflake-embryo-adoption Accessed April 2016.

28. Jean deBlois, Patrick Norris, and Kevin O'Rourke, *A Primer for Health Care Ethics Essays for a Pluralistic Society* (Washington, DC: Georgetown University Press, 1994).

29. Hastings Center Report, "When Baby's Mother Is Also Grandma and Sister," *Hastings Center Report* 15/5 (October 1985): 29.

30. Arthur L. Caplan, "The Ethics of In Vitro Fertilization," in *Ethical Issues in the New Reproductive Technologies,* ed. Richard T. Hull (Belmont, CA: Wadsworth, 1990).

31. Sambhu Charan Mondal, Anuradha Verma, Shiv Kumar Gupta, and Babita Kumar, "Genetic and Gestational Surrogacy: An Overview," *Walailak Journal of Science and Technology* 9/3 (2012): 189–93.

32. Birgitte, "*The Ethics of Surrogacy: A List of the Pros and Cons of Surrogacy.*" http://www.positive-parenting-ally.com/ethics-of-surrogacy.html. Accessed April 2016.

33. Rosalie Ber, "Ethical Issues in Gestational Surrogacy," *Theoretical Medicine and Bioethics* 21/2 (April 2000): 153–69.

34. Trevor Allis, "The Moral Implications of Motherhood by Hire," Issues in Medical Ethics 5/1 (1997): 21–2.

35. Ruth Macklin, "Is There Anything Wrong with Surrogate Motherhood? An Ethical Analysis," *Law, Medicine & Health Care* 16/1–2 (Spring/Summer 1988): 57–64.

36. Herbert T. Krimmel, "The Case against Surrogate Parenting," *Hastings Center Report* 13/5 (October 1983): 35–39.

37. Abigail Haworth, "*Womb for Rent: Surrogate Mothers in India.*" Reprinted from *Marie Claire* at http://www.webmd.com/infertility-and-reproduction/features/womb-rent-surrogate-mothers-india. Accessed April 2016.

38. Joanna Sugden and Aditi Malhotra, "Foreign Couples in Limbo After India Restricts Surrogacy Services," *The Wall Street Journal* November 16, 2015. http://www.wsj.com/articles/foreign-couples-in-limbo-after-india-restricts-surrogacy-services-1447698601. Accessed April 2016.

39. Elizabeth S. Anderson, "Is Woman's Labor a Commodity?" *Philosophy and Public Affairs* 19/1 (Winter 1990): 71–92.

Chapter 5

Genetics and Selective Reproduction

A landmark scientific enterprise of the late twentieth century was the *Human Genome Project* (HGP). Coordinated by the U.S. Department of Energy and the National Institutes of Health, this 13-year project had as goals the identification of all the genes in human DNA as well as determination of the sequences of the three billion chemical base pairs that make up human DNA. Although the HGP was completed in 2003, analyses of the data collected will continue for many years (1). This new knowledge "about the make-up and functioning of the chemical building blocks of human life will give rise to insights into the causes and pathways of numerous diseases that inflict untold suffering upon humanity," in turn "making possible opportunities for more effective diagnosis, prevention, and treatment of many diseases" (2).

Allied health professionals have already become involved in the realm of genetics in providing health care services. In fact, a field in allied health has emerged called the "genetic associate" (3, 4).

This chapter focuses on the interface of contemporary work in genetics and reproductive decision making.

Increasing knowledge of the genetic basis of various human traits coupled with medical technologies allow parents to engage in *selective reproduction,* choosing particular characteristics they want their future children to have or not to have.

In this chapter, you will learn about:

- Use of preimplantation genetic diagnosis (PGD) for selecting for or against traits in children;
- Sex selection for medical and nonmedical reasons;
- The phenomenon of designer babies.

Case Study

Jenny Edwards and Chanita Miller are both studying for a career as genetic associates. They are also good friends. One weekend, they decide to go see the movie *Gattaca* which is being shown as part of a science film festival at their college. One scene near the beginning of the film really catches their attention.

The scene begins with the birth of Vincent to Marie and Antonio. Vincent was conceived naturally and testing immediately after birth predicts that he will likely have serious physical and psychological problems: neurological condition, 60% probability; manic depression, 42% probability; attention deficit disorder, 89% probability; heart disorder, 99% probability. With an early fatal potential, his life expectancy is predicted to be 30.2 years.

Thus Marie and Antonio decide to use technology in having a second child. Marie's eggs and Antonio sperm are used to create embryos. In a lab they are informed that, after screening, they have two healthy male embryos and two healthy female embryos. They are told that these embryos have no critical predisposition to any major inheritable diseases. Marie and Antonio must now "select the most compatible candidate." First, they must decide on the gender of their child. They indicate that they would like to have a brother for Vincent to play with. They have already specified that they want their child to have hazel eyes, dark hair, and fair skin. In selecting embryos the lab has also eradicated any potentially prejudicial conditions such as baldness, myopia, alcoholism, addictiveness susceptibility, propensity to violence, and obesity. And so their second son Anton is born.

Jenny and Chanita leave the movie wondering whether what they have seen is science fiction or real life (5).

■ ■ ■

Preimplantation Genetic Diagnosis

This scene from *Gattaca* displays use of a technology that is currently available called *preimplantation genetic diagnosis (PGD)*. This procedure was originally developed to detect genetic disorders before a pregnancy begins. (6) The procedure typically begins with creating embryos through in vitro fertilization. The fertilized ova are allowed to develop to about the eight cell stage, at which time a cell is removed for genetic analysis. If a developing embryo is found to be free of the genetic disorder(s) for which it is being tested, it will be transferred to a woman's body to try to achieve a pregnancy. If an embryo is found to be affected by a genetic disorder, it will be discarded (6, 7, 8). In the scene from *Gattaca*, the embryos of Marie and Antonio were screened for predispositions to major inheritable diseases.

On the one hand, PGD is good for both the parents and the child in ensuring that a healthy child will be born. On the other hand, PGD involves disposing of embryos affected by a genetic disorder. From this perspective, whether PGD is judged an ethically permissible course of action depends on one's view of the status of the early stage embryo (see Chapter 3). If one believes that an embryo at the eight cell stage is not yet a human being, then one will not have any ethical qualms about disposing of the embryos affected by a genetic disorder. But if one believes that human life begins at conception/fertilization, one will see the disposal of the affected embryos as killing a human being and in the same category as abortion (8).

In so far as PGD is dependent on the creation of embryos through in vitro fertilization, previously noted concerns about IVF also apply to PGD (see Chapter 4). Further, from a practical point of view, the use of PGD does not guarantee that the procedure will result in a baby being born because embryo transfer has substantially less than a 100 percent success rate in achieving a pregnancy (6).

Ethically, PGD has been characterized as a form of unjust discrimination against persons with diseases or disabilities and as an affront to their human dignity (8). It has provoked negative reactions from persons with disabilities:

> Those in the disability community argue that identifying fetuses or embryos as candidates for termination or discard because they will, once born, have a disability, is equally vicious and destructively discriminatory. They maintain that the view that "fetal indications" justify termination or discard stems from the ignorant and prejudiced belief that having a disability makes life unbearable, and that those who are disabled are "better off unborn." Disability rights advocates maintain that disabilities are largely socially constructed. The appropriate response is to change society's attitude toward disability, not to try to get rid of disabled individuals. (9)

Indeed, some opponents of PGD has gone so far as to describe it as "the expression of a *eugenic mentality*" (8).

Sex Selection

In the scene from *Gattaca*, Marie and Antonio are presented with two male embryos and two female embryos. They are first asked to decide on the gender of their child. Marie responds that they would like a brother for their son Vincent to play with. Thus, they engage in sex selection of a male child.

There are two different reasons why parents might wish to select the sex of their child: medical reasons and parental preference.

In the first case, sex selection is used for the sake of the health of the child. There are sex-linked genetic diseases that only affect a child of one sex. Examples are Duchenne muscular dystrophy and hemophilia, both of which affect males (10, 11). Or again, some genetic disorders are more severely expressed in one gender than the other. Examples include Fragile X syndrome and autism. Parents who are carriers of such genetic diseases may wish to have children of the gender associated with a less severe form of the disease (10).

In the second case, parents simply prefer to have a child of a particular sex. In some instances, this preference is culturally influenced. For example, parents in parts of India may prefer sons because of the burden the dowry system imposes on the bride's family (12). Or again, in Western countries parents may engage in sex selection to achieve a "balanced family." One gender is already represented in the family and a child of the other gender is desired (10), or there may be an unequal representation of both genders among current siblings (13).

From an ethical point of view, there are two perspectives from which sex selection must be considered. One perspective is the ethical permissibility of the particular method used for sex selection. A second perspective is the ethical permissibility in principle of choosing the sex of our children.

Sex selection can occur postfertilization. Prenatal diagnosis can be undertaken to determine the sex of the fetus, followed by abortion of a fetus of the unwanted sex. (12) Or embryos can be created using in vitro fertilization (IVF) followed by determination of the sex of the embryos through PGD; PGD will also check the embryos for genetic abnormalities (13). A few of the normal embryos of the desired sex are then transferred to a woman to attempt a pregnancy (13). Remaining normal embryos may be frozen for later use, discarded, or donated for laboratory use. Embryos which are abnormal or unusable for any reason are discarded or donated for laboratory use (13). One's assessment of the ethical permissibility of these methods of sex selection is dependent on one's assessment of the ethical permissibility of abortion (see Chapter 3), on one's ethical assessment of IVF and the disposition of unused embryos (see Chapter 4), and on one's ethical assessment of PGD (see above).

A method of prefertilization sex selection is the MicroSort procedure developed and patented by the Genetics & IVF Institute in Fairfax, Virginia (14). This procedure separates X-bearing sperm (determining a female) from Y-bearing sperm (determining a male) by "staining the sperm with a fluorescent dye and then leading them past a laser beam where the difference in DNA content between X- and Y-bearing sperm gives a measurable difference in fluorescence" (12). Use of the X-sorted sperm has "led in 92% of the resulting pregnancies to a girl, whereas after the use of Y-sorted sperm, the result was a boy in 83.6%" (12). MicroSort can be used with intrauterine insemination (15). It can also be used in conjunction with IVF and PGD (15), in which case ethical assessment of the procedure becomes tied up with the ethical assessment of IVF and PGD.

The Genetics & IVF Institute set up a clinical trial with MicroSort with the aim of attaining FDA approval of this technology. The clinical trial was halted because of high costs and regulatory burdens. Consequently, the MicroSort technology is no longer available in the United States. However, MicroSort-licensed centers are available in Mexico, Northern Cyprus, and Switzerland (12).

It is widely agreed that use of sex selection for medical reasons (viz., to avoid genetic disease) is, in principle, acceptable (12). Ethical issues would center on the particular method used. On the other hand, use of sex selection for nonmedical reasons (i.e., parental preference) has been "the subject of recurrent ethical and public policy debate in many countries" (12).

Some would invoke the ethical principle of autonomy (see Chapter 1) in support of parental reproductive choice. In turn, "a common argument asserts that . . . choosing the sex of one's baby with available technology is part of a couple's basic right to reproductive choice" (16). In fact, sex selection is seen as a "logical extension of parents' rights to control the number, timing, spacing, and quality of their offspring" (16). Further, it is argued that sex selection for parental preference could "make a positive contribution to the quality of parent–child relationships, as children would not have to bear the burden of being wanted less because of their sex" (12). Further, parents may engage in sex selection for the sake of "family balancing," and it might be thought to be beneficial for the children themselves "to have the experience of growing up in a family of both boys and girls" (12).

On the other hand, there is concern that the practice of sex selection for parental preference will upset the male/female sex ratio in the population. In fact, "there is extensive evidence that the use of sex selection has resulted in significant disparities in child sex ratios in some South and East Asian countries, and in particular China and India" (17). While acknowledging this, it has been argued that the cultural climate in Europe and the United States is different and that "there is no reason to think that in Western countries, the wider availability of sex selection technologies will lead to a distortion of the sex ratio" (12). But it has also been pointed out that "there are many diaspora communities living in industrialized northern-hemisphere countries, some from cultures in which sex selection has been found to result in demographic imbalance" so that, "if sex selection were to be permitted in host countries, the possibility arises of such imbalance occurring in those countries, even if localized in specific communities" (17).

A major objection to sex selection for parental preference is that it embodies sexism in the sense of sex stereotyping (11). Typically, parents do not want a child of a particular sex because of biological features. For example, they do not desire a boy in order to have a child capable of strong beard growth (11). Rather, what they are aiming at in sex selection is character traits associated with a particular sex (11).

> Parents whose preference for one sex or another is compelling enough for them to take active steps to control the outcome must . . . be committed to certain strong gender-role expectations of the children they will raise. As sociologist Barbara Katz Rothman points out, the genetic test selects for sex, that is, for a child with XX or XY chromosomes, but what the parents are really selecting for is *gender*, the social role of being a boy or girl, man or woman. When people go out of their way to choose, they don't just want the right chromosomes and the attendant anatomical characteristics, they want a set of traits that go with "girlness or boyness." (16)

Concomitantly, parents who engage in sex selection of their children may force the child "into an unduly narrow or restrictive 'gender role' (boys made to fish and girls to shop . . .)" (11). Such parents are likely to "channel their children in certain directions" (11). Such parental attitudes violate a child's right to an "open future," that is, that a range of life plans be available to the child and that the child be able to choose among them without undue pressure from parents or society (11; see also 16).

Yet other potential harmful effects of sex selection for parental preference have been noted. If parents are able to choose what sort of children they are going to have, then parents may become less willing to tolerate their children's shortcomings (17). In turn, "the child's self-esteem could be adversely affected, undermining the unconditional acceptance of a child" (17).

Objection has also been raised to sex selection for parental preference from the perspective of Kantian ethics (see Chapter 1). Children "should be wanted and valued for their intrinsic worth as human beings" (17). Their value "should not be conditional on their possession of specific characteristics" such as being of a particular sex (17).

Finally, there is fear of a slippery slope effect. "If sex selection is accepted," it is argued, then "the next step will be selection to avoid short children, near-sighted children, or children whose intelligence is merely average" (16). We now turn to the potential expansion of traits parents could select in their children.

Selecting Embryos for Desired Traits

More and more, a genetic basis is being discovered for various human traits (18). This grounds the concept of *designer babies*, children born with improved genetic endowments through human design. A designer baby could be created through screening and selecting of embryos carrying desirable traits or through genetic changes being made in gametes or embryos (genetic engineering) (18).

In *Gattaca* PGD is used not only to eliminate embryos with negative traits (e.g., baldness, myopia, alcoholism, addictiveness susceptibility, propensity to violence, obesity) but to select embryos having positive traits desired by the parents (hazel eyes, dark hair, fair skin). The parents Marie and Antonio might also have used PGD to select in favor of their child having such desirable traits as increased IQ, perfect pitch, better memory, or increased longevity (18).

This use of PGD may seem attractive because parents typically "hope not only for healthy children, but for children best endowed to live fulfilling lives" (18). Ethically, it might be defended on the grounds of parental reproductive freedom (18). Since the child himself would presumably benefit from having the selected positive traits, the ethical principle of beneficence (see Chapter 2) might also be invoked in support of this use of PGD.

On the other hand, concern has been expressed that, "owing to the sheer expense of IVF and PGD . . . not all couples who could benefit from these procedures [would] have unfettered access to them" (18). In other words, access to this technology "might be a privilege enjoyed exclusively by the rich" (18). Socially, this could create a "genobility" (19). Society could be "divided between the economically *and* genetically rich, on the one hand, and the economically *and* genetically poor on the other" (18). Ethically, this concern falls under the principle of distributive justice (see Chapter 1).

It is also feared that the use of PGD to select for traits in children will significantly change the attitudes of parents toward their children:

The attitude of parents toward their child may be quietly shifted from unconditional acceptance to critical scrutiny: the very first act

of parenting now becomes not the unreserved welcoming of an arriving child, but the judging of his or her fitness, while still an embryo,
to become their child, all by the standards of contemporary genetic
screening. (18)

Indeed, human reproduction turns into "making a product to selected specifi-
cations" (18).

Selecting a child for certain desired traits inevitably creates "specific hopes
and expectations as to how their child might excel" (18). Thus the child must
"bear the burden of living up to the standards he was 'designed' to meet" (18).
These parental expectations "may impinge upon the child's freedom to make
his own way in the world" (18). Thus using PGD to select for parentally desired
traits in a child may be a mixed blessing for the child himself.

CHAPTER SUMMARY

Key Terms and Concepts

human genome project (HGP): a scientific project identifying all the genes in
human DNA and determining the sequences of the chemical base pairs
that make up human DNA.
preimplantation genetic diagnosis (PGD): a procedure for testing embryos for
specific genetically based traits prior to the embryo being transferred to a
woman to establish a pregnancy.
sex selection: use of methods aimed at achieving a child of a particular sex.
designer baby: use of technologies to achieve a child with particular traits.

Key Points

■ Preimplantation genetic diagnosis (PGD) was originally developed to screen
embryos for genetic disorders. Its use has been expanded to screen embryos
for non-medical traits.

■ The ethical evaluation of preimplantation genetic diagnosis involves the ethical evaluation of in vitro fertilization and of disposing of early stage embryos.

■ Because preimplantation genetic diagnosis selects against embryos with
genetic disorders, it has been accused of being a form of discrimination
against persons with diseases and disabilities.

■ There are two different reasons why parents may wish to select the sex of their child: medical reasons (e.g., to avoid a child being affected by a sex-linked genetic disorder) and parental preference (e.g., the desire to have a balanced family with children of both sexes).

■ The ethical assessment of sex selection involves the particular method used.

■ A major concern about practicing sex selection for parental preference is that it embodies sexism in the sense of sex stereotyping.

■ It is feared that increased use of PGD to select for desired traits in children will change the attitude of parents toward children from one of unconditional acceptance to critical scrutiny of the child's worthiness to be born. Concomitantly, such parental selection creates performance expectations for a child that may hamper his freedom to make his own way in the world.

FOR FURTHER DISCUSSION

1. Sarah and John Goldberg were married 3 months ago. Through a program at their synagogue they have learned that they belong to a population at risk for Tay-Sachs disease. An infant with this genetic disease appears to develop normally for the first few months of life. Then, as his or her nerve cells become distended with fatty material, a progressive mental and physical deterioration occurs. The child becomes blind, deaf, and unable to swallow, and muscles begin to atrophy with paralysis setting in. There is currently no cure for Tay-Sachs and, even with the best of care, children with this disease usually die by age 4 (20).

Tay-Sachs is a recessive inherited genetic disorder, so that a person must have two copies of the gene to have the disease. Someone can be a "carrier," having just one copy of the gene; in this case, the person will be unaffected by the disease. Both parents must be carriers of the gene for Tay-Sachs in order for a child to be affected by this disease. If both parents are carriers, there is a 25 percent chance for any pregnancy that the child will be affected by Tay-Sachs (20).

While Sarah and John dream of having several children, they definitely don't want any child of theirs to be afflicted with such a devastating disease as Tay-Sachs. For this reason, they decide to undergo the simple blood test that will determine if they are carriers. The worst case scenario occurs. They find out that they are both carriers for Tay-Sachs.

Unwilling to give up their dream of having children, Sarah and John make an appointment with a genetic counselor. The counselor tells them that they have the following options for having children:

- Take a chance and conceive a child naturally, but with the intent of accepting the child whatever his or her health condition.
- Conceive a child naturally but use prenatal diagnosis to determine the genetic status of the fetus, with the intent of aborting any fetus affected by Tay-Sachs.
- Use in vitro fertilization to produce embryos which will undergo PGD, using only those embryos not affected by Tay-Sachs to try to achieve a pregnancy.
- Use donor sperm or ova from someone who does not carry the gene for Tay-Sachs to conceive a child through artificial insemination or in vitro fertilization.
- Forgo having their own biological children and adopt.

Reflecting on the discussions in Chapters 3 and 4 as well as this chapter:

- *Are there any courses of action you would rule out as ethically impermissible? And why?*
- *Which course(s) of action do you regard as ethically permissible? What reasons can you give to support your judgment? If you consider a particular course of action to be ethically permissible, can you answer any ethical concerns that might be voiced about it?*
- *From practical and ethical points of view, which do you think is the best course of action for Sarah and John to take? And why?*

2. Suppose you learned that your parents had selected your sex. What would be your reaction? Suppose you learned that your parents had selected the sex of a younger brother or sister after they gave birth to you. What would be your reaction?
3. Parents who are deaf may use PGD to select children who will also be deaf. It is argued that deafness is not a handicap or disability but a variant on the spectrum of normalcy. Indeed, deaf people have their own rich culture and their own nonverbal sign language (21). From an ethical point of view, are there any problems with parents selecting in favor of a trait for their child which is generally regarded as a disability?

References

1. U.S. Department of Energy, "*Human Genome Project Information.*" http://www.ornl.gov/sci/techresources/Human_Genome/home.shtml. Accessed May 2016.

2. Catholic Health Association of the United States, *Facilitator's Resource Manual for Harnessing the Promise of Genomics* (St. Louis, MO: Catholic Health Association of the United States, 2004).

3. J.H. Marks and M.L. Richter, "The Genetic Associate: A New Health Professional," *American Journal of Public Health* 66/4 (1976): 388–90.

4. Thomas R. Mertens, Jon R. Hendrix, and Kathleen M. Kenkel, "The Genetic Associate: A Career Option in Genetic Counseling," *Journal of Heredity* 77/3 (May–June 1986): 175–78.

5. *Gattaca.* Columbia Pictures, 1997.

6. Human Fertilisation and Embryology Authority and Advisory Committee on Genetic Testing, *Consultation Document on Preimplantation Genetic Diagnosis.* http://www.hfea.gov.uk/cps/rde/xbcr/hfea/PGD_document.pdf. Accessed April 2016.

7. Ricki Lewis, *Human Genetics*, 5th ed. (New York: McGraw-Hill, 2003).

8. Vatican Congregation for the Doctrine of the Faith, *Instruction Dignitas Personae on Certain Bioethical Questions.* http://www.vatican.va/roman_curia/congregations/cfaith/documents/rc_con_cfaith_doc_20081208_dignitas-personae_en.html. Accessed April 2016.

9. Bonnie Steinbock, "Preimplantation Genetic Diagnosis and Embryo Selection," in *A Companion to Genethics,* ed. Justine Burley and John Harris (Malden, MA: Blackwell, 2004).

10. Center for Human Reproduction, *Gender Selection.* https://www.centerforhumanreprod.com/services/infertility-treatments/genderselection. Accessed April 2016.

11. Stephen Wilkinson, *Choosing Tomorrow's Children The Ethics of Selective Reproduction* (New York, NY: Oxford University Press, 2010).

12. European Society of Human Reproduction and Embryology Task Force on Ethics and Law, "Sex-Selection for Non-medical Reasons," *Human Reproduction* 28/6 (2013): 1448–54.

13. Genetics & IVF Institute, *Family Balancing.* http://www.givf.com/familybalancing. Accessed April 2016.

14. Center for Human Reproduction, *What MicroSort Tells Clinical Trial Participants.* https://www.centerforhumanreprod.com/fertility/what-microsort-tells-clinical-trial-participants. Accessed April 2016.

15. North Cyprus Fertility Clinic, *Gender Selection Options.* http://www.donasyon.net > Gender Selection Options. Accessed April 2016.

16. Dena S. Davis, *Genetic Dilemmas: Reproductive Technology, Parental Choices, and Children's Futures,* 2nd ed. (New York, NY: Oxford University Press, 2010).

17. Lucy Frith, "Ethical Objections to Sex Selection for Non-medical Reasons," *Reproductive BioMedicine Online* 16/1 (25 January 2008): 41–45.

18. President's Council on Bioethics, *Beyond Therapy Biotechnology and the Pursuit of Happiness* (Washington, DC: The President's Council on Bioethics, October 2003).

19. Ronald M. Green, *Babies by Design the Ethics of Genetic Choice* (New Haven, CT: Yale University Press, 2007).

20. National Institute of Neuorological Disorders and Stroke of the National Institutes of Health, *NINDS Tay-Sachs Disease Information Page*." http://www.ninds.nih.gov/disorders/taysachs/taysachs.htm. Accessed May 2016.

21. European Society of Human Reproduction and Embryology Task Force on Ethics and Law, "Preimplantation Genetic Diagnosis," *Human Reproduction* 29/8 (2014): 1610–17.

Chapter 6

Treatment Decisions for Seriously Ill Newborns

When parents await the birth of a child, what they have in mind is the birth of a normal, healthy child who is "cute and cuddly." But sometimes parents undergo the emotional trauma of having a child who has serious health problems. Infants can be born prematurely and with low birth weight. These infants can have problems with immature lung development, feeding, susceptibility to infections, internal hemorrhage, and anemia (1). Some infants are born with disabilities and even with life-threatening congenital abnormalities. In such cases, decisions must often be made whether to give medical treatments to the infant or withhold them.

In this chapter, you will learn about:

- Ethical principles for making decisions about using or withholding medical treatments in the case of seriously ill newborns;
- The scope of parental rights in treatment decision making for their children;
- The pros and cons of practicing euthanasia in the case of seriously ill newborns.

Case Study

Emilio Sanchez is a laboratory technician at a university medical center. Emilio usually does the lab work for the neonatal unit, and he knows the physicians and nursing staff in that unit quite well. During the last week there have been two especially difficult cases in that unit that have left Emilio wondering about the right thing to do for seriously ill newborns.

On Monday, Charles and Marilyn Birmingham had a son with anencephaly, a neural tube defect resulting in absence of a major portion of the brain (forebrain and cerebral cortex). A baby born with anencephaly is usually blind and deaf, unconscious, and unable to feel pain. There is no cure or standard treatment for anencephaly, and the prognosis for babies born with this condition is extremely poor. If the infant is not stillborn, the infant usually dies within a few hours or days after birth (2). After prenatal testing, the Birmingham's pediatrician had told them that their baby would be born with this condition, but they decided to carry the pregnancy to term anyway. In fact, Charles and Marilyn made it clear that, if the baby were born alive, they wanted the child placed in the neonatal intensive care unit and "everything possible done" to save the child's life. Their pediatrician had reluctantly agreed to their request. However, the nurses in the neonatal intensive care unit were very uncomfortable with this decision and felt that they were being asked to prolong the suffering of the child. They felt relieved when the child died a day and a half after birth.

The stress level for staff increased when Sarah Gordon gave birth to a baby girl with Down syndrome and, along with this, a digestive system blockage which prevents normal intake of food and liquids. Sarah's pediatrician assured her that the blockage could be surgically corrected and the sooner, the better. However, Sarah indicated that she wanted to allow the child to die. "My husband is unemployed and I am a student at a community college, and we're trying to get our own lives together," she stated. "We just couldn't deal with a special needs child. My parents live in another state and my husband's parents both have health problems, so they are not able to help us with caregiving. Besides, the intestinal blockage is nature's way of saying that the baby should not live. She'll be better off in heaven." The staff in the neonatal unit disagreed with the mother's decision and discussed whether they should seek a court appointed guardian for the baby girl to authorize the surgery. When Emilio Sanchez hears about this, he wonders, as an outsider, if they would be violating Sarah's rights as a parent in taking this course of action.

■ ■ ■

Focusing on the Welfare of the Child

In the second case, Sarah Gordon feels overwhelmed by the prospect of taking care of a child with special needs. The stress and hardship which can be involved with raising a seriously ill or disabled child have been described by a Hastings Center study group on imperiled newborns.

In addition to concerns about finances, a source of stress for parents is responsibility for home health care for the child (3). Parents "report that the demands on their energy and inner resources are high, and that some of them experience 'burn-out' over an extended period of time" with fatigue being "a major problem for families whose children require constant care" (3).

Families may also be stressed by fears about the future in terms of "the ambiguity that surrounds their child's future development and needs" and in terms of the availability of adequate services for their children at later points in time (3). They may face the possibility of a lifetime of responsibility for their child that will not be reduced as the child grows older (3).

Families may also experience feelings of social isolation and stigma (3). Neighbors may "object to having their child associate with the disabled child" (3). Some parents "are never able to go out together" because "one always has to be home to care for the child" (3).

Further, parental careers may be "attenuated and movement to suit employment limited" (3) On the other hand, parents who wish to remain at home to care for their children may be forced into the workplace "to meet the expenses of the child's treatments" (3).

However, some would point out that these hardships are not the whole story. Assistance is available to help parents and families cope with these difficulties. On a financial level, governmental assistance may be available to help with the cost of care (4). On an emotional level, "individual and group counseling can substantially alleviate anxiety, guilt, and frustration, and enable parents to cope with underlying conflicts triggered by the birth and the adaptation required" (4). Perhaps even more importantly, it has been pointed out that the experience of caring for a seriously ill or handicapped child can have a positive aspect to it:

> Finally, in many cases, the experience of living through a crisis is a deepening and enriching one, accelerating personality maturation, and giving a new sensitivity to the needs of spouse, siblings, and others. As one parent of a defective child states: "In the last months I have come closer to people and can understand them more. I have met them more deeply. I did not know there were so many people with troubles in the world". (4)

In sum, some would argue that "although we must recognize the burdens and frustrations" of raising an infant with health problems, "it does not necessarily follow that these costs require nontreatment" (4).

To ensure that the rights of seriously ill or disabled children are not compromised, some have recommended that treatment decisions for seriously ill newborns should focus almost exclusively on the welfare of the child himself. For example, the Council on Ethical and Judicial Affairs of the American Medical Association has taken the position that "the primary consideration for decisions regarding life-sustaining treatment for seriously ill newborns should be what is best for the newborn" (5). Similarly, the President's Commission for the Study of Ethical Problems in Medicine and Biomedical and Behavioral Research recommended that "parents should be able to choose among alternative treatments with similarly beneficial results and among providers, but not to reject treatment that is reliably expected to benefit a seriously ill newborn substantially. . . ." (1). Because "it is all too easy to undervalue the lives of handicapped infants," the Commission "excludes consideration of the negative effects of an impaired child's life on other persons, including parents, siblings, and society" (1).

Standards for Treatment Decision Making

Chapter 7, "Decisions about Using or Forgoing Life-Sustaining Treatments," will present the *principle of weighing benefits and burdens*, a widely accepted principle for making such decisions. This chapter will discuss other standards that have been proposed by ethicists specifically for the case of seriously ill newborns. These standards reflect a focus on the infant himself or herself. We will present three different standards developed by ethicists.

Medical Indications Policy   This standard focuses exclusively on the physical condition of the child. It directs that if a treatment is available that will work medically, it should be provided to the child. No infant should be denied medical treatments simply on the basis of his or her handicap or future quality of life. Treatment should be provided to all infants except when the infant is in the process of dying or when the treatment itself is medically inadvisable (3).

Best Interest of the Child   This standard allows the child's quality of life to be taken into account. It directs that an infant should be treated except when the infant is dying, or when the treatment itself is medically inadvisable, or when continued life would be worse for the child than an early death (3).

Relational Potential Standard   This standard is based on the belief that "the meaning, substance, and consummation of life is found in human relationships" (6). According to this standard, it is permissible to withhold medical treatments from an infant when the infant's potential for engaging in human relationships is simply nonexistent, or would be utterly submerged and undeveloped in the mere struggle to survive (6).

How do these standards apply to our case studies? First, how do these standards apply to the case of the Birmingham's anencephalic son? According to the medical indications policy, it would be permissible to forgo all life-sustaining treatments for the baby once it is born since the child can be regarded as in the process of dying; the prognosis for babies born with anencephaly is extremely poor, with such babies typically dying within a few hours or days after birth (2). The best interest standard also allows treatment to be forgone when an infant is dying. Similarly, the relational potential standard would justify withholding treatment from an anencephalic infant, although on different grounds: the absence of a cerebral cortex (the part of the brain primarily responsible for the psychological functions of consciousness, thought, and feeling) makes the child incapable of entering into characteristically human interrelationships (6). In sum, according to each of these principles, it is ethically justifiable to forgo life-sustaining treatments for the Birmingham's anencephalic son, as the nurses in the neonatal intensive care unit believe is best.

However, the case of Sarah Gordon's daughter with Down's syndrome and a digestive system blockage is different from an ethical point of view. According to the medical indications policy, the fact the child has the handicap of Down's syndrome and will not have a "normal life" is irrelevant to making the treatment decision. What should be considered are her physical condition (digestive system blockage) and whether there is a medical treatment available for this condition. The blockage is indeed a *treatable* condition through surgery; it is not the case that the child is in an irreversible process of dying. Further, the surgical repair of the digestive system blockage is medically advisable; in fact, the doctor thinks that the sooner the surgery is performed, the better. Therefore, according to the medical indications policy, Sarah's daughter should have this treatment.

The standard of the best interest of the child would consider all these factors, but would go beyond the requirements of the medical indications policy in also taking into account the child's quality of life. Here is one description of the life of Down's syndrome children:

> Developmental milestones (such as sitting, standing, and walking) come slowly, and toilet training may take several years. People with Down syndrome tend to have warm, loving personalities and enjoy art and music. Intelligence varies greatly, from those with profound mental retardation, to those who can follow simple directions, read, and use a computer. One young man with Down syndrome graduated from a junior college and another starred in a television series. (7)

At the present time, the degree of mental deficit that Sarah's daughter will suffer is not clear. This is one of the special challenges of making medical treatment decisions for newborns—the long-range outcome may be ambiguous or uncertain (1, 3). There is a real chance, however, that Sarah's daughter can have a quality of life that will make continued existence preferable to death. Thus, Sarah's daughter is not disqualified from receiving treatment according to the standard of the best interest of the child. This standard does not justify Sarah's decision to withhold the surgery from her daughter.

The relational potential standard for medical treatment decision making is different from the other two standards in making primary the ability of the child to enter into characteristically human relationships. By this standard, it is legitimate to withhold medical treatment under either of two conditions: (a) the child simply will not have the capability of entering into human relationships, or (b) so much time and effort would have to be devoted to mere physical survival that the child could not really cultivate human relationships. The description of Down's syndrome children indicates that many can enter into characteristically human relationships. They have "warm, loving personalities." They can share art and music with other people. They can participate in society by holding certain levels of jobs. Only if a Down's syndrome child was very severely mentally challenged or had some other overwhelming physical problem might it be questionable that the child could pass the relational potential standard for receiving medical treatment. In the case of Sarah's daughter, the digestive system blockage can be surgically repaired. The degree of mental deficit she will suffer is not clear at this point. Thus, Sarah's daughter is not disqualified from receiving medical treatment using the relational potential standard. Again, this standard does not justify withholding the surgery to correct the digestive system blockage.

Which of these three standards ought to be adopted as the principle for making medical treatment decisions in the case of seriously ill newborns? The answer may depend in part on one's conception of the purpose of health care and on other values one holds. Is the purpose of health care merely to address physical needs, or to address physical needs as a means of enabling a person to achieve a certain level of function and quality of life? Is existence and life on the physical plane intrinsically valuable? Or is such existence valuable only as enabling a person to engage in certain sorts of activities? And if we take into account quality of life considerations in making decisions about giving or forgoing medical treatments for newborns, can we ever get beyond such judgments being highly subjective and reflective of personal biases? (8)

Who Should Make the Treatment Decision?

In the second case, the nurses in the neonatal unit disagree with Sarah Gordon's decision to deny surgery for her infant daughter. They are contemplating going to court to get someone appointed as the baby's legal guardian who will authorize the surgery to be performed. Emilio Sanchez, the laboratory technician for the neonatal unit, wonders whether they would be violating Sarah's rights as a parent in taking this course of action. Ethically and legally, there is a presumption in favor of parental decision-making authority in the case of seriously ill newborns. Ethically, this stance is "rooted in the strong ties of affection and concern that parents have for their offspring," which means that "parents will endeavor to formulate decisions about medical care in accordance with their child's best interest" (3). Further, parents play an ongoing role in overseeing the lives of their children, and thus the law "recognizes that parents, to be parents, must be accorded the right to make basic decisions as to the welfare of their children" (3).

At the same time, "parents may be reeling emotionally from the shock of having a seriously ill child instead of the normal, healthy infant they had imagined" (1). They may be poorly informed about the child's medical condition and long-term prognosis (1). In these situations, health care providers can serve as advisors to parents, helping them "in sorting through possible treatment options and their consequences" (3).

Ideally, treatment decisions should be made jointly by parents and health care providers, and agreed upon by both. Nevertheless, cases may arise where parents reject treatment for a child that health care providers view as clearly effective, or insist on treatment that health care providers see as futile or harmful (3). In such situations, health care staff may call upon the resources of an ethics committee or an infant care review committee to assist in resolving the conflict (5; see Chapter 2).

Should an ethics consult not succeed in reconciling the views of parents and health care providers, legal recourse is available. As persons unable to protect themselves, infants fall under the *parens patriae* power of the government (1). In the exercise of this power, the state can override parental decisions to ensure that the child is not neglected or abused. The state's perceptions of what is in the interest of the child can take precedence over the views and decisions of parents (1).

In the case of Sarah Gordon and her daughter, the hospital nurses see Sarah as acting against her daughter's interests in denying her the surgery that would allow normal intake of food and liquids. Legally, they can go to court to try to override Sarah's decision.

In sum, while there is a presumption in favor of parental decision-making authority in the case of seriously ill newborns, it is also recognized that particular parents may not make reasonable decisions, and that parental authority over their children is not absolute.

Euthanasia in the Case of Seriously Ill Newborns

Thus far we have focused on the issue of forgoing life-sustaining treatments for seriously ill newborns. Some would go even farther and allow euthanasia for (at least some) seriously ill newborns. If abortion is permitted, why draw the line at birth for the permissibility of killing? After all, newborns seem closer to unborn fetuses than to adults (3). Moreover, once a decision is made not to use life-sustaining treatments, an earlier death through euthanasia may mean less suffering for the infant since sometimes an infant does not die immediately when life support is withdrawn or withheld (3).

For example, infants falling into the following category have been proposed as candidates for euthanasia:

> . . . there are infants with a hopeless prognosis who experience what parents and medical experts deem to be unbearable suffering. Although

it is difficult to define in the abstract, this group includes patients who are not dependent on intensive medical treatment but for whom a very poor quality of life, associated with sustained suffering, is predicted. For example, a child with the most serious form of spina bifida will have an extremely poor quality of life, even after many operations. This group also includes infants who have survived thanks to intensive care but for whom it becomes clear after intensive treatment has been completed that the quality of life will be very poor and for whom there is no hope of improvement (9).

Named after a university medical center in the Netherlands, the *Groningen Protocol* would allow euthanasia of such infants when five criteria are met:

- The infant's diagnosis and prognosis must be certain.
- The infant must be experiencing hopeless and unbearable suffering.
- At least one independent physician must confirm that the first two conditions are met.
- Both parents must give their informed consent.
- The termination procedure must be performed in accord with the accepted medical standard (10).

Needless to say, the concept of euthanasia for seriously ill infants has proven very controversial.

The Hastings Center study group on imperiled newborns raised several concerns about allowing infanticide as a matter of social policy. For one thing, health care professionals are fallible human beings, so that errors can occur in the prognosis given for a newborn and medical conditions can be misidentified. Further, if euthanasia were allowed for newborns, abuses could occur. Some parents could advocate killing their infants to serve their own purposes rather than their infants' welfare. Individual physicians may have strong feelings about particular kinds of disabilities being "worse than death" and so push the option of euthanasia. Hospitals may see opportunities to cut cost through the practice of euthanasia (3). Moreover, in response to the argument that dying infants will suffer in the absence of euthanasia, it can be pointed out that "advances in pain management make it possible to relieve all or almost all pain" (3).

For these reasons, the Hastings Center study group recommended that social policy should *not* permit the active killing of seriously ill and disabled infants (3).

CHAPTER SUMMARY

Key Terms and Concepts

medical indications policy: a principle specifically for treatment decision making in the case of seriously ill newborns that maintains that no infant should be denied medical treatments simply on the basis of his or her handicap or future quality of life. Treatment should be provided to all infants except when the infant is in the process of dying or when the treatment itself is medically inadvisable.

best interest of the child: a principle specifically for treatment decision making in the case of seriously ill newborns that maintains that infants should be treated except when the infant is dying, or when the treatment itself is medically inadvisable, or when continued life would be worse for the child than an early death.

relational potential standard: a principle specifically for treatment decision making in the case of seriously ill newborns that maintains the permissibility of withholding medical treatments from an infant when the infant's potential for engaging in human relationships is simply nonexistent or would be utterly submerged and undeveloped in the mere struggle to survive.

parens patriae power: a governmental power pertaining to persons who are unable to protect themselves, such as children, allowing the government to override parental decisions in order to ensure that the child is not neglected or abused.

Key Points

- There are hardships involved in caring for and raising a child with a serious illness or with a disability. At the same time, assistance is available to parents and families to cope with these difficulties. There can be positive, enriching aspects to the experience of caring for a seriously ill or handicapped child.
- To safeguard the interests and rights of the child, decisions about medical treatment for seriously ill newborns should focus on the welfare of the child himself or herself.
- Several standards have been proposed for medical treatment decision making specifically in the case of seriously ill newborns: the medical indications policy, the best interest of the child, and the relational potential standard.
- There is a presumption in favor of parental decision-making authority in the

case of seriously ill newborns. However, it is recognized that particular parents may not make reasonable decisions so that, legally, parental authority is not absolute. The court system has the power to override parental decisions to ensure that the child is not neglected or abused.

■ Some argue for the practice of euthanasia in the case of seriously ill newborns as an extension of the legally accepted practice of abortion and in order to provide a quick end to the infant's suffering. Opponents of euthanasia are concerned about errors being made in the prognosis for an infant, and about possible abuses of the practice of euthanasia. In addition, it is pointed out that good pain management can relieve the suffering of seriously ill newborns as they die.

FOR FURTHER DISCUSSION

1. Has anyone in your family or someone else you know suffered from a disease or disability since birth? How do you see the quality and value of their lives? How do they assess the quality and value of their lives?

2. Three different principles were presented for making treatment decisions in the case of seriously ill newborns: the medical indications policy, the principle of the best interest of the child, and the relational potential standard. Which of these principles do you personally favor for use in making treatment decisions for seriously ill newborns? Why?

3. A policy statement on *Treatment Decisions for Seriously Ill Newborns* formulated by the Council on Ethical and Judicial Affairs of the American Medical Association includes the following directives:

   The primary consideration for decisions regarding life-sustaining treatment for seriously ill newborns should be what is best for the newborn. Factors that should be weighed are (1) the chance that the therapy will succeed, (2) the risks involved with treatment and nontreatment, (3) the degree to which the therapy, if successful, will extend life, (4) the pain and discomfort associated with the therapy, and (5) the anticipated quality of life for the newborn with and without treatment.

   Care must be taken to evaluate the newborn's expected quality of life from the child's perspective. Life-sustaining treatment may be withheld or withdrawn from a newborn when the pain and suffering expected to be endured by the child will overwhelm any potential joy during his or her life. When an infant suffers extreme neurological damage, and is consequently not capable of experiencing either suffering or joy, a decision may be made to withhold or withdraw life-sustaining treatment. When life-sustaining treatment is withheld or withdrawn, comfort care must not be discontinued (5).

■ *Compare and contrast these directives with the principles presented in this chapter; namely, the medical indications policy, the principle of the best interest of the child, and the relational potential standard.*

■ *If these directives were used to guide the treatment decision in the case of the Birmingham's anencephalic son, what decision would be made?*

■ *If these directives were used to guide the treatment decision in the case of Sarah Gordon's daughter born with Down's syndrome and a digestive system blockage, what decision would be made?*

4. The authors of the Groningen Protocol propose that infants suffering from the most serious form of spina bifida are candidates for euthanasia (9). Do some background research on spina bifida. After learning the facts about spina bifida in its various forms, do you think that it is ever appropriate to forgo medical treatments for an infant suffering from spina bifida? Do you agree that infants suffering from the most serious form of spina bifida deserve euthanasia?

References

1. President's Commission for the Study of Ethical Problems in Medicine and Biomedical and Behavioral Research, *Deciding to Forego Life-Sustaining Treatment* (March 1983; reprint New York: Concern for Dying).
2. National Institute of Neurological Disorders and Stroke, *Anencephaly Information Page,* http://www.ninds.nih.gov/disorders/anencephaly/anencephaly.htmAccessed March 2016.
3. Arthur Caplan and Cynthia B. Cohen (eds.), "Imperiled Newborns," Hastings Center Project Report, Hastings *Center Report* 17/6 (December 1987): 5-31.
4. John A. Robertson, "Involuntary Euthanasia of Defective Newborns: A Legal Analysis," *Stanford Law Review* 27 (1975): 246-61.
5. Council on Ethical and Judicial Affairs of the American Medical Association, AMA's Code of Medical Ethics *Opinion* 2.215. http://www.ama-assn.org/ama/pub/physician-resources/medical-ethics/code-medical-ethics/opinion2215.page? Accessed March 2016.

6. Richard McCormick, S.J., "To Save or Let Die The Dilemma of Modern Medicine," *Journal of the American Medical Association* 229/2 (July 8, 1974): 172-76.

7. Ricki Lewis, *Human Genetics: Concepts and Applications,* 2nd ed. (Dubuque, IA: Wm. C. Brown, 1997).

8. Sadath A. Sayeed and Geoffrey Miller, "The Forgoing of Life-Sustaining Treatment for Children" in Geoffrey Miller (ed.), *Pediatric Bioethics* (New York: Cambridge University Press, 2010), pp. 262-83.

9. Eduard Verhagen and Pieter J.J. Sauer, "The Groningen Protocol— Euthanasia in Severely Ill Newborns," *New England Journal of Medicine* 352/10 (March 10, 2005): 959-62.

10. James Lemuel Smith, "The Groningen Protocol: The Why and the What" in Ronald Munson, *Intervention and Reflection Basic Issues in Medical Ethics,* 8th ed. (Belmont, CA: Thomson Wadsworth, 2008).

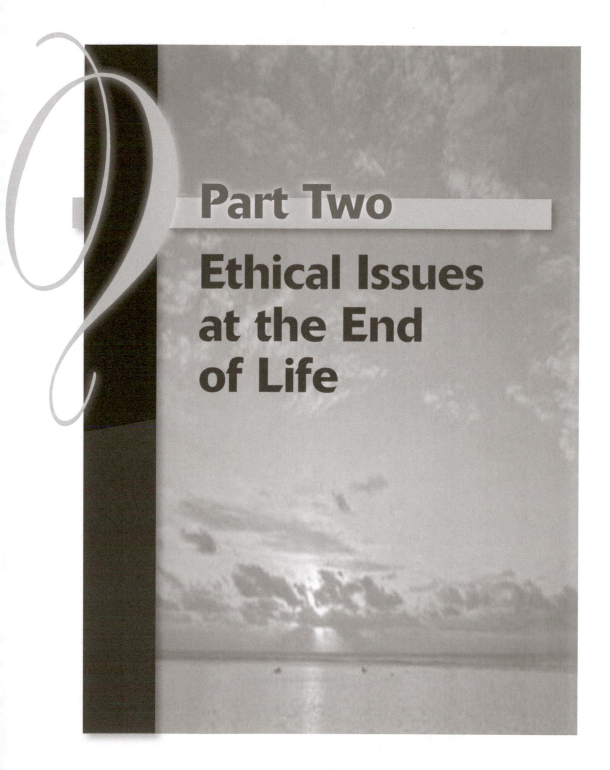

Part Two

Ethical Issues at the End of Life

Chapter 7

Making Decisions About Using or Forgoing Life-Sustaining Treatments

A *life-sustaining treatment* is "any medical intervention, technology, procedure, or medication that is administered to a patient in order to forestall the moment of death, whether or not the treatment is intended to affect the underlying life-threatening disease(s) or biologic processes" (1). Examples of life-sustaining treatments include chemotherapy, kidney dialysis, resuscitation, the use of a ventilator, and tube feeding. The administration of antibiotics or blood pressure medication can also fall into this category in some cases.

In this chapter, you will learn about:

- How to make decisions about using or forgoing life-sustaining treatments;
- Whether it is permissible to withdraw a treatment once it has been started;

95

- The difference between forgoing a life-sustaining treatment and euthanasia;
- Controversies concerning futile care.

Case Study

Roger and Kate Smith, both 76, have been residents of the Oak Park Home, a multilevel facility, for a year. Three years ago Roger had a cancerous tumor in his stomach, but chemotherapy had worked in shrinking it and causing the cancer to go into remission. However, within the last month, the cancer has recurred.

Chemotherapy is promptly begun for Roger. However, Roger's doctor is honest with him that, this time around, the chemotherapy will probably slow the growth of the tumor and prolong his life but is not likely to "cure" his cancer as it did before.

The first time Ray had cancer, he had tolerated the chemotherapy treatments reasonably well. But this time he experiences nausea and vomiting, and feels so "washed out" for a week after each treatment that he cannot even enjoy his grandchildren when they come to visit him. In addition, the pain from the cancer is considerable.

To make things worse, 2 months later Roger develops pneumonia. Because of his overall weakened physical condition, Roger's physician recommends hospitalization with antibiotic treatment and supplemental oxygen therapy. Initially, Roger agrees.

However, after 5 days in the hospital Roger writes a note to his respiratory therapist, Sue Martin, indicating that he no longer wants these treatments for his pneumonia. In fact, he indicates to his wife and his physician that he wants to stop chemotherapy treatments as well. All these treatments, he feels, are only prolonging his suffering. He states that he has lived a full life, and is ready to die. Roger had been a very successful attorney, and no one doubts that he is still sharp mentally.

Roger's wife Kate is sometimes at the hospital when Sue Martin looks in on Roger. In conversations with Kate, Sue learns that Roger and Kate have three children and that two of the children support Roger's decision to forgo all medical treatments while his wife Kate and one of their daughters disagree. They feel that Roger has "given up too soon." After all, he beat the odds with cancer once before, and he has grandchildren to live for and enjoy.

Sue knows that, if a decision is made to stop all medical treatments as Roger wishes, she will be involved in stopping the supplemental oxygen support. The conflict that exists within Roger's family makes Sue herself wonder what the right thing to do really is.

■ ■ ■

Ethical Principles for Making Decisions about Life-Sustaining Treatments

Two ethical principles are commonly brought into discussions about using or forgoing life-sustaining treatments: the *principle of autonomy* and the *principle of weighing benefits and burdens.*

Autonomy refers to self-determination, to directing the course of one's own life. Patient autonomy entails that a competent patient has a right to be involved in decision making about medical treatments, and indeed, to make the final decision about using or forgoing treatments (see Chapter 1).

In the case of Roger Smith, there is no doubt that he is "still sharp mentally," and thus competent to make medical treatment decisions. Roger has clearly expressed his desire to stop all the medical treatments being administered. According to the principle of autonomy, Roger's health care providers should agree to Ralph's wishes to stop chemotherapy treatments, the administration of antibiotics, and supplemental oxygen therapy.

Sometimes the principle of patient autonomy is presented in such a way that health care providers are expected to abide by the wishes of the patient no matter what he wants and no matter what the rationale for his decision. Experience with putting the principle of autonomy into practice is causing us to recognize certain limitations to patient choices. One of these limitations is the expectation that patients should make their treatment decisions in accord with accepted principles of health care ethics.

Historically, a distinction was made between *ordinary* and *extraordinary* medical treatments. The accompanying moral principle stated that ordinary treatments must always be provided when needed but there is no obligation to use treatments that are extraordinary (2, 3). Aspirin, blood pressure medication, and antibiotics might be considered ordinary treatments. Ventilators, chemotherapy, and kidney dialysis might be given as examples of extraordinary treatments. However, ethicists came to see problems with this distinction and the accompanying moral principle. Recently, ethicists have refined it into a *principle of weighing benefits and burdens.* This is not a completely new standard. Rather, it is an attempt to introduce clarity and precision into discussions by focusing on one of the traditional interpretations of the ordinary/extraordinary treatment distinction (2, 3).

The principle of weighing benefits and burdens sets out the following criteria for making decisions about using or forgoing life-sustaining treatments:

- If a treatment provides more benefits than burdens from the patient's perspective, the treatment should be provided.
- If the burdens of a treatment outweigh its benefits from the patient's perspective, it is permissible to forgo (i.e., withhold or withdraw) the treatment.
- If a treatment is useless or futile, not providing benefit to the patient, it is permissible to forgo (i.e., withhold or withdraw) the treatment (1–3).

The first criterion is supported by the principle of beneficence, and the second by the principle of nonmaleficence. The cases falling under the third criterion fail to satisfy the principle of beneficence, making it permissible to forgo the treatment.

If it is unclear whether the benefits or burdens of a treatment are greater, a time-limited trial of the treatment is appropriate in cases where this is practically possible for the particular type of treatment (4). In a time-limited trial, "an intervention is started with the prior understanding that after a defined period, the desirability of continuing the treatment will be reassessed" (4). Such a trial period "can help assess the benefits and burdens of a treatment if these are difficult to assess in advance" (4). From an ethical point of view, it is "preferable to try a treatment and to withdraw it if it fails, than to not try it at all" (1). On the one hand, "not starting [a treatment] in these circumstances could deprive the patient of beneficial treatment that the patient might find desirable" (1). On the other hand, a trial period can "help a patient or loved ones to be at peace with a subsequent decision to withdraw treatment" (4).

What is meant by the "benefits" a treatment might bring? For example, will the treatment bring about a cure (or even a partial cure) for the patient? Will it give the patient the opportunity to live longer? Will it give the patient relief from pain? Will it increase the patient's physical mobility? Will it restore the patient's consciousness? Will it enhance the patient's ability to communicate with family and friends? Will the consequences of the treatment give the patient the opportunity to do things that have meaning for him or her or give pleasure to him or her, or provide the patient with the possibility of fulfilling specific goals? (3, 4).

On the other hand, how can a treatment be "burdensome"? For example, will the treatment itself cause physical pain or suffering for the patient? Will the treatment entail any psychological burdens, such as depression? Will the treatment require that the patient expend a great amount of effort? (e.g., will the patient have to drive a substantial distance each week to get the treatment?) Will the patient have to be restrained to tolerate the treatment? (e.g., will the patient have to be restrained to prevent him from pulling out a feeding tube?) Does the patient have an intense fear of the treatment or a strong repugnance to it? Will the consequences of the treatment diminish the patient's ability to do things that have meaning for him or her or give him or her pleasure? Will the treatment impose a financial burden on the patient or his family? (3, 4, –5). These are examples of benefits and burdens of treatments, not an exhaustive list.

The principle of weighing benefits and burdens requires us to engage in something like a cost–benefit analysis. Balancing the sides, are the benefits of the treatment greater than the burdens? If the answer is yes, then the treatment should be undertaken. On the other hand, are the burdens greater than the benefits? Then it is morally permissible to forgo the treatment. Since individual patients may evaluate the benefits and burdens of a treatment differently, promoting the patient's good entails that benefits and burdens should be assessed *from the perspective of the particular patient* (1).

It should be noted that our interpretation of the principle of weighing benefits and burdens includes benefits and burdens both for the patient (e.g., increasing the patient's physical mobility) and for other people (e.g., the cost of the treatment for the patient's family). It also includes benefits and burdens of both a purely medical nature (e.g., physical pain and suffering caused by the treatment) and a nonmedical nature (e.g., the cost of treatment). What is more controversial is the inclusion of quality of life considerations. Should we limit ourselves to consideration of the burdensomeness *of the treatment itself,* or should we consider the burdensomeness *of the life sustained* through a treatment? (2). For example, pneumonia used to be called "the old person's friend" because it could bring about death for persons suffering from other debilitating diseases (6, 7). When assessing benefits and burdens, some ethicists advocate looking at "the well-being of the whole person" and not merely at the benefits of treatment to a particular organ (5). On this view, a medical intervention (such as dialysis) may replace a patient's kidney function but, given the patient's overall medical condition, may not really be a benefit to the patient (5).

In some cases, a treatment simply will not work physically for a patient. For example, some patients cannot tolerate tube feeding because the fluid would be too much for a weakened heart (8). Or again, antibiotics are ineffective against viral (vs. bacterial) pneumonia (9). In such cases, the particular treatment provides no benefit whatever to the patient. The principle of weighing benefits and burdens recognizes that when a treatment is useless or futile, there is no ethical obligation to use it.

When using the principle of weighing benefits and burdens to make decisions about life-sustaining treatments, decisions are made on a case-by-case basis. There is no treatment which must automatically be used. Similarly, there is no treatment which can automatically be forgone. The question to ask is: What will this treatment do for this particular patient who is in this particular condition? Even if a treatment is commonly available (such as antibiotics), there is not necessarily a moral obligation to use it (1).

In discussing life-sustaining treatments, we have spoken of both the principle of patient autonomy and the principle of weighing benefits and burdens. Is there a way of putting them together? While we should abide by the wishes of the patient, it is also true that patients should not make their decisions in a purely arbitrary way. We should encourage them and help them to look at the relative benefits and burdens of the treatment, and to make their decision on that basis.

How does all of this apply to the case of Roger Smith? First, do the benefits and burdens of the chemotherapy justify stopping this treatment? The chemotherapy is not expected to cure Roger's cancer. It is expected to slow the growth of the tumor and hence to prolong Roger's life, although we do not know for how long a time. Thus, while there is some benefit to Roger from the chemotherapy, the benefit is limited. On the other hand, the chemotherapy has some definitely burdensome aspects to it. Roger is experiencing nausea and vomiting from the chemotherapy, and treatments leave him feeling so "washed out" for a whole week that he cannot even enjoy his grandchildren when they come to visit him. Further, the pain Roger is experiencing from the cancer is considerable, and prolonging his life through administration of chemotherapy is only prolonging his suffering. In addition, there are the costs of continued aggressive treatment to consider, not only the chemotherapy treatments themselves but the fact that Roger must be placed in a unit of the Oak Park Home which provides a higher level of nursing care and hence is more expensive. Roger may worry about what will happen to his wife Kate if their financial resources are depleted. In sum, in this case it would be reasonable to judge that the burdens of Roger's chemotherapy treatments outweigh the benefits, and thus stopping the chemotherapy treatments is an ethically permissible course of action.

Patients who are terminally ill with cancer are prone to infections (10, 11, 12). This has happened to Roger in developing pneumonia Antibiotics are routinely administered for infections, and it is often assumed that administering antibiotics is invariably beneficial (1). However, burdens can be associated with the use of antibiotics. The side effects of antibiotics can include nausea, diarrhea, the risk of *Clostridium difficile* infection, bleeding due to impaired vitamin K, and drug resistance (4, 13).

The method of administering antibiotics can also be burdensome in some respects, for example, repeated injections and the increasing difficult search for suitable injection sites, and maintaining intravenous lines (1, 10, 14). Thus, weighing benefits and burdens cannot be ignored when dealing with antibiotics for a particular patient (13, 15).

In considering the benefits and burdens of antibiotic treatment for Roger, his rationale for wanting to stop all medical treatments is noteworthy. Roger states that he has lived a full life, is ready to die, and that the medical treatments are only prolonging his suffering. In the case of patients who are terminally ill and contract an infection, a major argument for forgoing the use of antibiotics is that the temporary prolongation of life provided by curing the infection is only prolonging the suffering of the dying process (1):

> Those incremental increases [in length of life] come at the risk of increased distress as the underlying chronic disease progresses with increased symptoms. These elements can compound patient distress at the end of life and multiply both patient and family suffering. (14)

In other words, in these circumstances "any treatment that extends life, no matter how simple the treatment is, offers more burden than benefit" (7).

However, there is another factor to consider before deeming it ethically permissible for Roger to forgo the antibiotic treatment. Even when a decision has been made to forgo life-sustaining treatments for a patient, it is still considered ethically obligatory to provide comfort care for the patient (1). Can antibiotics provide Roger with the important benefit of comfort care and be obligatory to provide on this basis? In some cases, antibiotics can palliate symptoms, as in the case of a patient suffering with a symptomatic urinary tract infection, and should be provided (12, 13, 14). However, for many types of pneumonia, there are more effective symptom management techniques than antibiotics, such as opioids and antipyretics (12, 13, 14). Thus, even if Roger forgoes chemotherapy and antibiotics, these types of medications are appropriately provided for him as comfort care. The same holds true for the supplemental oxygen therapy being given to Roger. If this therapy makes it more comfortable for him to breathe, it should be continued.

Misconceptions about Forgoing Life-Sustaining Treatments

The case of Roger Smith involves stopping chemotherapy. In the past, some have made a distinction between *withholding* a life-sustaining treatment (i.e., never starting a treatment) and *withdrawing* a treatment (i.e., stopping a treatment). Some judged that it is morally permissible to withhold a treatment but that, once started, a treatment cannot be stopped (1). This kind of thinking has changed. Ethically, it is now considered just as permissible to withdraw a treatment as never to start it (1). It may be more difficult emotionally and psychologically for family members or health care workers to stop a treatment than never to start it. But if we have tried a treatment and then decide to withdraw it for lack of beneficial results, we can at least feel that we have done everything we can to help the patient (1).

Some family members or health care workers may feel guilty about withdrawing a life-sustaining treatment. The reason is that they feel they will be doing something to cause the death of the patient. In other words, they are afraid that, in stopping a life-sustaining treatment, they will be engaging in an act of euthanasia. This fear is unfounded. Daniel Callahan clearly distinguishes euthanasia ("killing") from forgoing a life-sustaining treatment ("letting die") in terms of what is the *cause of death* and in terms of the *intention* behind the action:

> . . . as a reality of nature, killing and letting die are causally different. "Letting die" is only physically possible if there is some underlying disease that will serve as the cause of death. Put me on a respirator now, when I am in good health, and nothing whatever will happen if it is turned off. I cannot be "allowed to die" by having a respirator turned off if I have healthy lungs. It is wholly different, however, if a doctor gives me a muscle-relaxing injection that will paralyze my lungs. Healthy or not, those lungs will cease to function and I will die. That is what it means to "kill" someone as distinguished from "letting someone die." Put more formally, there must be an underlying fatal pathology if allowing to die is even possible. Nothing but the action of the doctor giving the lethal injection is necessary to bring about death.
>
> . . . Here is Rachels' second mistake: to assume that the intention in letting die is ordinarily the same as in killing, that is, to make a person dead. It is certainly the case that we *might* intend someone's death and turn off a machine to bring that about. But it is equally the case . . . that patients are allowed to die because of a judgment that it no longer makes sense, medically or morally or both, to continue life-extending treatment. Doctors have long stopped treating patients when their skills and art run out. There is no reason to think that, as a rule, it is because their intentional goal is to make people die. (16)

In sum, in the case of forgoing a life-sustaining treatment, there is an underlying fatal pathology which made the use of the life-sustaining treatment necessary in the first place and which will be the direct cause of the patient's death when the treatment is stopped. Further, the direct intent in withdrawing a life-sustaining treatment is not to end the life of the patient, but to stop a treatment that is no longer justified medically or morally.

Another misconception about decisions to forgo life-sustaining treatment is that, once such a decision has been made, the patient will simply be abandoned by health care providers. This is not true. Pain medication and comfort care will still be provided. A slogan has surfaced in health care, "Care, not cure" (17). A time may come in a patient's illness when nothing more can be done medically to help the patient recover from the disease. At this stage the emphasis changes to one of relieving the symptoms of the disease and of enabling the patient to spend his final days in as comfortable and meaningful a way as possible.

Finally, if a decision has been made to stop treatment, this does not mean that the treatment must be withdrawn immediately. Time can be provided for family members and friends to say final good byes and for religious rituals to take place before the treatment is stopped and the patient is allowed to die.

Case Study

Elaine Manion, 28, has been battling cystic fibrosis (CF) since birth. In spite of the daily therapy needed to clear her lungs, she has tried to stay active and live as normal a life as possible. She has become the manager of a restaurant, and teaches religious education classes to children in her church. Elaine knows that people with CF have a shortened life span, and that she is nearing the maximum life expectancy for persons with CF.

As Elaine nears her 29th birthday, her health begins to fail. She is repeatedly hospitalized. For several years Elaine has been working closely with Michael Adams, a respiratory therapist, and Jane Finnegan, a physical therapist who provides postural drainage therapy. Both Michael and Jane recognize that Elaine has begun the "final downhill slide."

During her latest hospitalization, Elaine's doctor, Marilyn Lee, advises her to have a Do-Not-Resuscitate (DNR) order. A cardiopulmonary arrest, Dr. Lee says, would simply be a part of her body giving out in the dying process. Cardiopulmonary resuscitation (CPR) might not work at all in restoring her heart beat and respiration and, even if it did, Elaine would likely suffer another arrest in a few days.

Elaine, however, refuses to consent to a DNR order. She believes that God can work miracles for those who believe in him. In Elaine's view, declining to forgo resuscitation—just standing by and allowing death to come— would show a lack of faith in God's power to heal. Elaine repeatedly tells Dr. Lee and her therapists that she wants all available treatments, including resuscitation.

Dr. Lee feels strongly that resuscitation would be "futile" in Elaine's case. She is tempted to simply write a DNR order on Elaine's chart. This is a case, she believes, in which "the doctor knows best" and the patient is acting irrationally. Michael Adams agrees with Dr. Lee, but Jane Finnegan isn't so sure. After all, shouldn't health care providers first and foremost respect a patient's wishes?

■ ■ ■

The Question of Medical Futility

According to the principle of weighing benefits and burdens, it is permissible to forgo a life-sustaining treatment that is futile. Suppose, however, that a patient (or family member) wants, or even demands, a treatment that health care providers regard as futile. From an ethical point of view, should the treatment be provided?

The ethical principle of autonomy might be brought forward as an argument for an affirmative answer (18, 19). This principle entails that it is the right of a patient (or his or her proxy decision maker) to make the ultimate decision about medical treatments (see Chapter 1). On the other hand, it is argued that it is irresponsible and a violation of professional integrity for a health care professional to offer or provide a therapy that is unlikely to work (20, 21). Further, such action may offer false hope to a patient (19) or even increase a patient's pain and discomfort in the final days of life (22). On this view, patient autonomy is meaningful only when the patient is presented with a choice between medically viable options, and futile treatment is not really a viable option (21, 23, 24). In sum:

Although the ethical requirement to respect patient autonomy entitles a patient to choose from among medically acceptable treatment options (or to reject all options), it does not entitle patients to receive whatever treatments they ask for. Instead, the obligations of physicians are limited to offering treatments that are consistent with professional standards of care (22).

The last statement could be expanded beyond physicians to any health care professional.

Another dimension of the futility dilemma is determining exactly what constitutes "futile" treatment. How should medical futility be defined? The answer is surprisingly complex.

On an intuitive level, medical futility "refers to interventions that are unlikely to produce any significant benefit for the patient" (22). But how narrowly or how broadly should "benefit" for the patient be understood? In this regard, we find it useful to distinguish definitions of futility which take a *physicalist* approach from those, which take a *personalist* approach.

Physicalist definitions of futility focus on the body of a patient and physiological outcomes of medical interventions. For example:

- A medical intervention is futile if the patient has a lethal diagnosis or prognosis of imminent death (18).
- A medical intervention is futile if evidence exists that the intervention cannot achieve its physiologic goal (18).
- A medical intervention is futile if the intervention does not work in more than 1 percent of attempts (25) or, otherwise stated, if it is ineffective more than 99 percent of the time (20).
- A medical intervention is futile if evidence exists that the intervention will not or cannot extend the patient's life span (18).

Concomitantly, a medical intervention would not be considered futile if undertaken for a patient who does not have a lethal diagnosis or who is not imminently dying. Or again, a medical intervention would not be considered futile if it can achieve its physiologic goal; for example, if resuscitation will, in fact, revive a patient. The third definition is a statistical specification of the second (18).

On the fourth definition, an intervention would not be considered futile if it had the benefit of extending a patient's life span, although what constitutes an enhanced life span is ambiguous (viz., a day, a week, a month) (18)

Personalist definitions of futility consider the broader context of a patient's life, considering not merely the patient's body but "the patient as person" (19). For example:

- A medical intervention is futile if evidence exists that the intervention will not or cannot enhance the patient's quality of life (18).
- A medical intervention is futile if evidence exists that the intervention will not or cannot achieve the patient's or family's goals (18).

For example, a medical intervention might prolong a patient's life (and, on a physicalist understanding of futility, not be futile treatment) but leave the patient incapable of surviving outside the intensive care unit. From a quality of life perspective, this could be considered futile treatment (19). On the other hand, suppose that a woman who has ovarian cancer and who is close to death would like to reconcile with an estranged son before she dies. And let us suppose further that she develops pneumonia. From a physicalist perspective, using antibiotics to treat her pneumonia might be judged futile treatment on the grounds that she is imminently dying. However, if treating her with antibiotics will buy a few days' time and allow her to achieve the personal goal of seeing her son, then this medical intervention would not be considered futile treatment from a personalist perspective. In sum, the various definitions of futility can yield different judgments about the futility of a medical intervention for a particular patient.

Which definition of futility should be adopted? The Council on Ethical and Judicial Affairs of the American Medical Association has taken the position that "futility is intrinsically a value judgment" and hence found "great difficulty in assigning an absolute definition to the term futile care" (25). Instead, the Council proposed a process for decision making in cases of apparent futility, a process which can be generalized beyond physicians:

- Earnest attempts should be made in advance to deliberate over and negotiate prior understandings between patient, proxy and physician on what constitutes futile care for the patient, and what falls within acceptable limits for the physician, family, and possibly also the institution.
- Joint decision making should occur between patient or proxy and physician to the maximum extent possible.
- Attempts should be made to negotiate disagreements if they arise, and to reach resolution within all parties' acceptable limits, with the assistance of consultants as appropriate.
- Involvement of an institutional committee, such as the ethics committee should be requested if disagreements are irresolvable.
- If the institutional review supports the patient's position and the physician remains unpersuaded, transfer of care to another physician within the institution may be arranged.
- If the process supports the physician's position and the patient/proxy remains unpersuaded, transfer to another institution may be sought and, if done, should be supported by the transferring and receiving institution.
- If transfer is not possible the intervention need not be offered (25).

Noteworthy is the role assigned to an ethics committee in dealing with disputes about futility (see Chapter 2). The process outlined "allows a hearing for patient and proxy assessments of worthwhile outcome" as well as for consideration of the perspectives of health care providers (25). It is preferable to unilateral decision making on the part of a health care professional to deny a treatment which, from his or her point of view, is futile (18). This process also has the advantage of providing a system for addressing ethical dilemmas regarding futility without the need for recourse to the court system (25).

CHAPTER SUMMARY

Key Terms and Concepts

principle of patient autonomy: self-determination; an individual's right to hold views, make choices, and take actions based on personal values and beliefs.

principle of weighing benefits and burdens: A life-sustaining treatment ought to be used if it provides more benefits than burdens. It is morally permissible to forgo (i.e., withhold or withdraw) a life-sustaining treatment if the burdens of the treatment outweigh its benefits or if the treatment is useless or futile.

Key Points

- Patients themselves, not health care providers, have the right to make the final decision about using or forgoing life-sustaining treatments (principle of patient autonomy).
- Patients should make their decisions on the basis of considering the relative benefits and burdens of the treatment (principle of weighing benefits and burdens).
- It is ethically permissible either to *withhold* or to *withdraw* a life-sustaining treatment.
- Withholding or withdrawing a life-sustaining treatment is *not* the same as euthanasia.
- It is ethically permissible to withhold or withdraw a treatment that is futile. Problems arise from the fact that different people understand "futility" in different ways.

FOR FURTHER DISCUSSION

1. Have you ever experienced in your family or with close friends a situation in which a decision had to be made about using or forgoing life-sustaining treatments? Describe the case and the decision that was made. Why was this particular decision made? If the decision were up to you, would you have made the same decision or a different one? Why or why not?

2. The case of Roger Smith presented in this chapter represents a situation of family conflict regarding the use of life-sustaining treatments. Roger, the patient in question, wishes to forgo all medical treatments, and two of his children support him in making this choice. On the other hand, Roger's wife Kate and one of their daughters disagree with Roger's decision.

   In American medical ethics, a good deal of emphasis is placed on patient autonomy. Following this principle, it would be concluded that health care providers should do what Roger wants, even if family members cannot accept his decision. Some contend, however, that an exclusive emphasis on patient autonomy represents an extreme form of individualism that ignores the fact that we are involved in relationships with other people and that our actions as individuals also affect them.

   In your view, should Roger's wife and children have any say in the decision about using or forgoing medical treatments? If so, what do you think their appropriate role is? Do you think that the ethical principle of autonomy should be limited in any way?

3. As a result of an automobile accident 4 months ago, Martha Miller, 54, is paralyzed from the waist down and must use a wheel chair for mobility. Since being released from the hospital, an occupational therapist, Ted Marlow, has been working with Martha to evaluate her home environment and to recommend adaptations. Martha is divorced and her two adult children live out of state, but Ted is confident that Martha will be able to live independently and even be able to continue her work as a journalist out of her home.

   However, Martha's adjustment to her new situation is complicated by the fact that she develops kidney problems. Her physician recommends starting dialysis treatment, and indicates that her prognosis is good for living at least 10 more years if she begins dialysis immediately. The local Dial-a-Ride service can provide transportation for Martha to the dialysis center.

   Martha tells her physician that "enough is enough" and that she just wants to be left alone.

The physician is concerned that Martha is acting out of depression, and asks for a consult with the ethics committee at the local hospital to seek guidance in handling this situation. The physician asks Ted Marlow to participate in the ethics consult as one of Martha's caregivers.

Role-play this ethics consult. Have participants assume the roles of ethics committee members, Martha's physician, Ted Marlow the occupational therapist, and Martha Miller herself.

- *Supose that Martha is persuaded to attend the ethics consult meeting. How might she explain and justify her decision to forgo dialysis?*
- *Suppose you are Martha's physician. How might you argue in favor of Martha undertaking dialysis?*
- *Suppose that you are Ted Marlow, the occupational therapist working with Martha. As an "outsider," how do you see Martha's desire to forgo the dialysis treatment?*
- *What ethical principles should be brought forward by the members of the ethics committee to guide decision making in this case? How do these principles apply to this case? What facts about this case are important in applying these principles?*

After considering these various points of view and the ethical principles for making decisions about life-sustaining treatments, do you personally think that Martha should undertake dialysis or not? What factors in the case do you consider critical in coming to this judgment?

4. Consider the case of Elaine Manion presented in this chapter. Dr. Lee considers resuscitation to be "futile" treatment in her case. What concept(s) of futility might underlie Dr. Lee's judgment? Could any case be made that an attempt to resuscitate Elaine should not be considered "futile" treatment? In your judgment, should an attempt to resuscitate Elaine be considered "futile" treatment?

References

1. Hastings Center, *Guidelines on the Termination of Life-Sustaining Treatment and the Care of the Dying* (Briarcliff Manor, NY: Hastings Center, 1987).
2. President's Commission for the Study of Ethical Problems in Medicine and Biomedical and Behavioral Research, *Deciding to Forego Life-Sustaining Treatment* (New York, NY: Concern for Dying, 1983; reprint).

3. Benedict M. Ashley, O.P., Jean deBlois, C.S.J., and Kevin D. O'Rourke, O.P., *Health Care Ethics A Catholic Theological Analysis,* 5th ed. (Washington, DC: Georgetown University Press, 2006).

4. Nancy Berlinger, Bruce Jennings, and Susan W. Wolf, *The Hastings Center Guidelines for Decisions on Life-Sustaining Treatment and Care Near the End of Life,* 2nd ed. (New York: Oxford University Press, 2013).

5. Catholic Health Association of the United States, *Caring for People at the End of Life.* End-of-Life Guides (2015). https://www.chaus.org "Publications" Books and Printed Resources in the CHA Stores. Accessed January 2016.

6. Hank Dunn, *Hard Choices for Loving People* (Herndon, VA: A&A Publishers, 2001). https://www.stjosephhospicefoundation.org/images/pdfs/HardChoices.pdf. Accessed January 2016.

7. Esther-Lee Marcus, A. Mark Clarfield, and Allon E. Moses, "Ethical Issues Relating to the Use of Antimicrobial Therapy in Older Adults," *Clinical Infectious Diseases* 33/10 (2001): 1697–1705.

8. Joanne Lynn and James F. Childress, "Must Patients Always Be Given Food and Water?" in *By No Extraordinary Means: The Choice to Forgo Life-Sustaining Food and Water,* ed. Joanne Lynn (Bloomington, IN: Indiana University Press, 1986).

9. Healthline, *Pneumonia,* http://www.healthline.com/health/pneumonia. Accessed January 2016.

10. Stephanie Nagy-Agren and Harold B. Haley, "Management of Infections in Palliative Care Patients With Advanced Cancer," *Journal of Pain and Symptom Management* 24/1 (July 2002): 64–70.

11. An-Hsuan Chih, Long-Teng Lee, Shao-Yi Cheng, Chien-An Yao, Wen-Yu Hu, Ching-Yu Chen, and Tai-Yuan Chiu, "Is It Appropriate to Withdraw Antibics in Terminal Patients With Cancer With Infection," *Journal of Palliative Medicine* 16/11 (2013): 1417–22.

12. Adis Medical Writers, "In Patients Receiving End-of-Life Care, Medications Used to Treat Co-morbid Diseases Should Be Discontinued When Appropriate," *Drugs & Therapy Perspectives* 30 (2014): 432–34.

13. Robert E. Enck, "Antibiotic Use In End-of-Life Care: A Soft Line?" *American Journal of Hospice & Palliative Medicine* 27/4 (2010): 237–38.

14. Paul J. Ford, Thomas G. Fraser, Mellar P. Davis, and Eric Kodish, "Anti-Infective Therapy at End of Life: Ethical Decision-Making in Hospice-Eligible Patients," *Bioethics* 19/4 (2005): 379–92.

15. Erin Diviney Chun, Phillip E. Rodgers, Caroline A. Vitale, Curtis D. Collins, and Preeti N. Malani, "Antimicrobial Use Among Patients Receiving Palliative Care Consultation," *American Journal of Hospice & Palliative Medicine* 27/4 (2010): 261–65.

16. Daniel Callahan, *The Troubled Dream of Life in Search of a Peaceful Death* (New York, NY: Simon & Schuster, 1993).

17. Mary Sawyer, "Care, Not Cure: What to Say When Treatment Fails," *Journal of Hospice and Palliative Nursing* 4/3 (July/September 2002): 133–35.

18. Committee on Ethics of the American College of Obstetricians and Gynecologists, *ACOG Committee Opinion: Medical Futility* (March 2007; reaffirmed 2015), http://www.acog.org/Resources_And-Publications/Committee-Opinions/Committee-on-Ethics/Medical-Futility. Accessed January 2016.

19. Lawrence J. Schneiderman, Nancy S. Jecker, and Albert R. Jonsen, "Medical Futility: Response to Critiques," *Annals of Internal Medicine* 125/8 (15 October 1996): 669–74.

20. Endlink Resource for End of Life Care Education, *Definitions of Medical Futility*, http://endlink.lurie.northwestern.edu/eolc_medical_futility.cfm. Accessed January 2016.

21. Tom Tomlinson and Howard Brody, "Futility and the Ethics of Resuscitation," *Journal of the American Medical Association* 264/10 (September 12, 1990): 1276–80.

22. Nancy S. Jecker, "Futility," in *Ethics in Medicine University of Washington School of Medicine* (1998). http://depts.washington.edu/bioethx/topics/futil.html. Accessed January 2009.

23. James Drane and John Coulehan, "The Concept of Futility: Patients Do Not Have a Right to Demand Medically Useless Treatment," *Health Progress* 74/10 (December 1993): 28–32.

24. Marcia Angell, "The Case of Helga Wanglie: A New Kind of 'Right to Die' Case," *New England Journal of Medicine* 325 (1991): 511–12.

25. Council on Ethical and Judicial Affairs of the American Medical Association, *Opinion 2.037 Medical Futility in End-of-Life Care.* http://www.ama-assn.org/ama/pub/physician-resources/medical-ethics/code-medical-ethics.page 2.00 Opinions on Social Policy Issues. Accessed January 2016.

Chapter 8

Proxy Decision Making and Advance Directives

Patient Roger Smith (Chapter 7) is still able to make his own health care decisions. But suppose that, in addition to cancer and pneumonia, Roger was also suffering from dementia. Who should make the decisions about continuing or discontinuing chemotherapy and about providing or refusing the doctor's recommended treatments for pneumonia? And on what basis should these decisions be made?

These questions lead to consideration of advance directives. An *advance directive* is a legal document in which an individual makes provision for future medical treatment decisions in the event that he or she loses decision-making capacity. There are two basic types of advance directive: the *living will* and the *durable power of attorney for health care.* These documents may be called by various names in different states.

In this chapter, you will learn:

- Who can serve as a proxy decision maker;
- How a proxy should make treatment decisions;
- What a living will says and when it goes into effect;
- What a durable power of attorney for health care does and how it differs from a living will;
- How to execute advance directives;
- What requirements for advance directives are set by federal law;
- The advantages of having advance directives;
- Challenges in using advance directives;
- Types of advance care planning other than traditional advance directives.

Case Study

Mel Langley taught math for 20 years at Elkader Community College before taking early retirement 2 years ago. Since his retirement, Mel has remained so active that his friends from the college joke that he has "flunked retirement." Mel is an avid reader, checking out a new set of books from the library every week. He has resumed playing the piano, something he had to give up because of the time demands of his job. He is a regular volunteer at the local senior center, and continues to tutor students in math at the college. During the summer, he travels around the country attending Elderhostel programs.

Recently, Jim Parker, Mel's friend who also taught math at the college, was diagnosed with cancer. Over a period of a year, Mel visits Jim twice a week. Mel watches Jim suffering from chemotherapy treatments and undergo repeated hospitalization. His weight loss is significant. At Jim's funeral, Mel comments that Jim doesn't even "look like himself" any more.

Jim's death causes Mel to wonder what would happen if he should be diagnosed with a terminal illness. In order to protect himself against lingering in a debilitated condition, Mel decides to make out advance directives—both a living will and a durable power of attorney for health care document. Mel never married, but he has two sisters and a younger brother. Mel names his brother as his proxy decision maker in executing his advance directives.

One Sunday morning while attending church services, Mel begins to experience severe chest pains. He is taken to the emergency room of the local hospital, where he is diagnosed as having suffered a fairly severe heart attack.

During his stay in the cardiac care unit of the hospital, Mel is given a thorough physical. It is discovered that he has prostate cancer. Mel's physician, Dr. Reynolds, thinks the condition is curable with radiation therapy. He contacts Barbara O'Connor, a radiation therapist at the hospital, to inquire when Mel could be fit into the hospital's radiation therapy program.

Medications being administered to Mel for his heart condition have left him confused, and Dr. Reynolds does not think that he has the capacity at this point to make sound decisions about his health care. For this reason, Dr. Reynolds contacts Mel's brother to authorize the treatment for prostate cancer. Dr. Reynolds wants to begin the treatment regimen as soon as Mel is stronger.

To Dr. Reynolds' surprise, his brother produces Mel's advance directives and says that nothing should be done for Mel's prostate cancer. He even raises the possibility of having Mel discharged from the cardiac care unit and taken home to die. "Mel would never want to live like this," his brother states, "where he can no longer do what he used to enjoy."

Dr. Reynolds does not agree with Mel's brother. He does not think that Mel is "at the brink of death." To be sure, Mel's heart problems will leave him with a more restricted life style, but that is not the same as being terminally ill. And his prostate cancer is very likely curable.

Mel's two sisters also come to see him, and approach Dr. Reynolds about his prognosis. They too disagree with the judgment of Mel's brother. At this point, they feel everything possible should be done to save Mel's life.

Dr. Reynolds decides to arrange a meeting with Mel's brother and two sisters to try to resolve the dispute. He invites Barbara O'Connor to attend in order to help explain the projected radiation therapy to Mel's family.

Barbara has recently completed her training in radiation therapy and is a new employee at the hospital. She has heard about the conflicts that can occur between physicians and family members over treatment decisions, and among members of the same family. This is the first time she has personally witnessed a conflict where a patient's very life is at stake. She wonders who is right, and how the advance directives will play out in this situation.

■ ■ ■

Proxy Decision Making

First of all, the case of Mel Langley represents a situation in which someone other than the patient must be called upon to make the medical treatment decisions because the patient himself is presently suffering from confusion due to his medications. Someone who makes health care decisions for a patient who is not mentally competent to do so is referred to as a *proxy (or surrogate) decision maker.*

This role is often assumed by the patient's next of kin, but another relative, or a close friend, or an individual who knows the patient well may serve in this capacity. Often one of these individuals naturally emerges as the proxy decision maker. For example, if Mel were married, it would be natural for his wife to be called upon to make treatment decisions on his behalf. However, it is also possible for a patient to go beyond these informal arrangements and to select in advance an individual who will be legally recognized as his proxy decision maker. This is done by executing the legal document known as a *durable power of attorney for health care* (or as a *medical power of attorney*). In our case scenario, Mel Langley executed this document and legally named his younger brother as his proxy decision maker. If a patient has not executed this document, it is possible for a court to appoint a guardian to serve legally as the patient's proxy decision maker.

From an ethical point of view, how should a proxy decision maker go about making his decision on behalf of the patient? The preferred standard for proxy decision making is *substituted judgment.* According to this standard, the proxy decision maker attempts to reach the decision that the incapacitated person would make if he or she were able to choose (1). Thus, the proxy decision maker is guided by any explicit directives given by the patient, in writing or orally in conversation (2). If the patient has not left any explicit directives about the treatment in question, the proxy applies what is known about the patient's beliefs, values, preferences, and life-long behavior patterns to try to determine what the patient would have wanted (2).

There are some cases in which the principle of substituted judgment cannot be applied. This is so if the patient has never been mentally competent during his lifetime and thus was never able to express any preferences. This is also the case if the patient never in fact expressed any views about the treatment in question and no longer has any close living relatives or friends who know him well enough to make predictions about his wishes. In such cases, the *best interests standard* may be used. According to this standard, the proxy decision maker tries "to make a choice for the patient that seeks to implement what is in that person's best interests by reference to more objective, societally shared criteria" (1). This standard "does not rest on the value of self-determination but solely on protection of patients' welfare" (1). It is sometimes expressed as choosing as a reasonable person in the patient's circumstances would (2).

It is important to keep in mind that substituted judgment is the preferred standard for proxy decision making whenever it can be used. Making decisions in accord with the wishes and values of the patient represents an extension of patient autonomy to cases in which a patient cannot directly say what she wants.

The Living Will

In applying the standard of substituted judgment, a proxy decision maker should look first to any instructions the patient has made explicit in writing through the execution of advance directives.

The first type of advance directive that was developed is the living will. A living will typically applies to a patient who is *terminally ill* (3, 4); it might also be specified that the patient is *expected to die within a short period of time* (5). The condition of *permanent unconsciousness* may also be included in the scope of the living will (6, 7). A living will basically says that the patient does not want life-sustaining treatments used in these circumstances. In such cases, life-sustaining treatments would not help improve the condition of the patient, but would only prolong the dying process. However, comfort care and pain medication will still be provided to the patient.

Some people are afraid to sign a living will because they think they will automatically be denied treatment in the case of any medical emergency. This is not true. For example, if someone with a living will is in a car accident and is taken to the hospital emergency room and can recover, this document will not prevent her from receiving treatment to aid in the recovery.

It is important to keep in mind that a living will goes into effect only when an individual no longer has the capacity to make his own decisions. If someone is in the dying process but is conscious and lucid, he should still be asked directly what he does and does not want done in terms of medical treatments.

Durable Power of Attorney for Health Care

Because of limitations in the living will, another form of advance directive was developed, namely, the durable power of attorney for health care.

The language of a living will document usually gives only general directives about life-sustaining treatments. When signing such a document, an individual cannot foresee all the particular conditions which will prevail when the use of life-sustaining treatments becomes an issue in his own case. In order to provide for better decision making, a durable power of attorney for health care allows an individual to designate legally someone to make treatment decisions on his behalf when he is no longer able to do so. The legally designated proxy can engage in give-and-take discussion of medical alternatives. It is also possible to designate someone as an alternate proxy decision maker should the designated proxy be unavailable at the time a treatment decision must be made.

The durable power of attorney for health care is broader in scope than a living will. It goes into effect in any situation in which the patient becomes incapable of making treatment decisions, even temporarily. It is not limited to cases in which someone is terminally ill or permanently unconscious. Suppose that an individual—let's call him Jerome—has executed this document naming his wife Beth as his legal proxy. And suppose that Jerome gets into a car accident, suffers a concussion and broken ribs, and is taken to the hospital unconscious. Beth will have the legal authority to make any needed treatment decisions on Jerome's behalf. And when Jerome regains consciousness and decision-making capacity, the right to make treatment decisions will go back to him.

The person designated as the proxy decision maker through a durable power of attorney for health care *legally* has the right to make treatment decisions and even takes precedence over (other) relatives of the patient. Many families are not aware of this. The designated proxy may (and probably should) consult with the patient's (other) relatives to try to achieve agreement on the course of action to be taken. However, the designated proxy legally has the final say about what happens.

A durable power of attorney for health care document may include a space in which the person executing the document may write in instructions about specific treatments that he does or does not want in a particular circumstance; for example, instructions about resuscitation, dialysis, chemotherapy, antibiotics, or assisted nutrition and hydration. The designated proxy is expected to act in accord with such instructions.

It is also important to keep in mind that a durable power of attorney for health care is a different legal document than a power of attorney for financial matters. The individual designated to take care of someone else's finances does *not* automatically have the power to make medical decisions for that individual.

Executing Advance Directives

A living will or a durable power of attorney for health care can only be executed by someone who is mentally competent and of legal age to do so. An adult suffering from dementia who has not already executed an advance directive can no longer do so. Similarly, adults who have suffered from severe mental deficiencies since birth cannot execute advance directives.

A person can only execute an advance directive for himself or herself. So, for example, a wife cannot execute an advance directive for a husband suffering from dementia. A parent cannot execute an advance directive for a son or daughter, even for an adult child who is incapacitated and being cared for by the parents. In such cases, a court may be asked to officially appoint a relative (or another person) as *guardian* of the patient to make treatment decisions for the patient, or often family members close to the patient simply make such decisions. It is not absolutely necessary to see a lawyer to execute a living will or durable power of attorney for health care. Health care facilities have individuals on staff trained to provide assistance in making out these documents, usually in social services or pastoral care.

At the present time, there is no federal legislation establishing the living will and durable power of attorney for health care for the entire United States, or establishing a standard form for executing them. Legally, these documents have been established state by state. Basically, the content of them is the same, but there may be differences among various states on such matters as who may witness the document, notarization rather than witnessing, or restrictions on who may be named as the proxy decision maker. In some states, individuals may be required to give explicit directions about assisted nutrition and hydration or about treatment in a condition of permanent unconsciousness.

Thus, the question arises of whether an advance directive written in one state will be recognized in other states. The Commission on Legal Problems of the Elderly of the American Bar Association has given this response:

> Many states expressly recognize out-of-state advance directives if the directive meets either the legal requirements of the state where executed or the state where the treatment decision arises. Several states are silent on this question. If there is doubt, the rules of the state where treatment takes place, not the state where the advance directive was signed, will normally control. (8)

The Commission advises that "even if an advance directive fails to meet technicalities of state law, health providers still should value the directive as important, if not controlling, evidence of the patient's wishes" (8).

While the original of an advance directive should be kept in a safe place, advance directives are not meant to be hidden. Copies of advance directives should be given to the patient's physician, family members, and proxy decision maker. The provisions of these documents should be discussed with them so that they feel comfortable with the instructions about treatment. It is also good to give a copy of advance directives to the hospital the person uses to have on record in the event of admission. Copies should also be provided to other health care facilities and services the patient is using (e.g., a nursing home or hospice program). It may also be a good idea to give copies to close friends and neighbors, since these are sometimes the first individuals to find someone at home undergoing a health care crisis. Some people also keep a reduced size photocopy of their advance directives in their wallets.

Advance directives are not just for senior citizens. They are useful for any adult to have. In fact, several well-known court cases about the withdrawal of life-sustaining treatments—the cases of Karen Ann Quinlan, Nancy Cruzan, and Terri Schiavo—involved young adults in their 20s and 30s! (9).

Advance directive documents can be changed or even revoked. They should be reviewed periodically to ensure that they still reflect the wishes of the person who has executed them.

The Patient Self-Determination Act

Federal legislation, called the *Patient Self-Determination Act,* has established requirements regarding advance directives for health care providers receiving Medicare and/or Medicaid funding. Specifically, the legislation sets the following requirements:

- A health care facility or agency must provide written information to each adult concerning his or her rights under state law to make decisions concerning medical care. This should include information about the right to accept or refuse medical or surgical treatment and the right to formulate advance directives.
- A health care facility or service must have written policies respecting the implementation of these rights.
- A health care facility or service must inquire in the case of each adult whether she has an advance directive.
- Documentation must be made in the patient's medical record whether he has executed an advance directive.
- A health care facility or service cannot condition the provision of care or otherwise discriminate against an individual based on whether she has executed an advance directive.
- A health care facility or service must comply with the requirements of state laws respecting advance directives.

- Health care facilities and services must provide education on advance directives for staff and for the community at large (10).

The law does *not* require a health care facility or agency to carry out any directive whatever contained in a living will or durable power of attorney for health care. No facility or agency is required to act contrary to its mission and ethical values, even if a patient requests this in writing. However, a facility or service must provide written policies specifying the limits on the procedures it will perform. And a clear summary of the facility's or service's policies regarding advance directives and consent to or refusal of medical treatment must be available to the public (10).

It is very important to recognize that the Patient Self-Determination Act does *not* require anyone to execute advance directives, but only requires that patients be informed that these documents are available for their use.

Finally, health care workers may be required to attend in-service programs on advance directives. Such educational programs for the staff of a health care facility or service are mandated by the Patient Self-Determination Act (10).

Advantages of Advance Directives

Autonomy (self-determination) is a value much emphasized in health care today. Advance directives are a way of extending the ethical value of patient autonomy. They allow a patient to control medical treatment decision making when she no longer has the ability to state her wishes directly. Advance directives are also regarded as a way of preventing the overuse of life-sustaining treatments. People may have seen the lives of family members and friends prolonged in a much debilitated state, and their response is, "I would never want that to happen to me!" Indeed, in the case scenario of Mel Langley, it is Mel's experience of a friend dying of cancer that prompts him to execute advance directives.

We live in a litigious society. Health care providers may sometimes be reluctant to withhold or withdraw life-sustaining treatments for fear of being legally liable. However, if an advance directive has been executed and the health care provider acts in accord with it in not providing life-sustaining treatments, the health care provider has protection (11). Thus, advance directives can make health care providers more comfortable about complying with requests to forgo life-sustaining treatments.

Advance directives can also be useful when conflicts arise among family members or between family members and health care providers. In such circumstances, if a durable power of attorney for health care has been executed, the designated proxy legally has the power to make the final decision and bring the conflict to resolution. Executing advance directives can prevent conflicts from going to court for resolution.

Challenges in Using Advance Directives

Through a living will, an individual indicates a desire to forgo life-sustaining treatments when terminally ill or permanently unconscious. An individual may also give directions about types of treatments that are or are not wanted in a variety of circumstances in a durable power of attorney for health care document. But can anyone accurately predict how she will *feel* in such circumstances? For example, when a person is healthy and active, she may view life with a serious, debilitating illness as unacceptable. But when she is actually in such a condition, holding on to life may appear very different. (For example, what is your own reaction to the possibility of suffering an accident that would leave you a quadriplegic in a wheelchair? And might you change your mind if this actually happened to you?)

Another problem concerns how to write instructions included in advance directives. Let's suppose that someone—let's call him Ben—has prepared advance directives stipulating that "under no circumstances" does he want to be hooked up to a breathing machine "for any illness." And let's further suppose that Ben subsequently suffers from delirium and Guillain–Barré syndrome (a potentially reversible illness causing progressive weakness and paralysis) and that Ben's physician recommends to his wife, Thelma, that he be placed on a ventilator, telling her that there is a 60 percent chance of full recovery with temporary ventilator support. Thelma knows the instructions Ben gave in his advance directives. She also believes that, when Ben gave these instructions, he thought that being connected to a ventilator meant that he would merely have biological functioning sustained indefinitely with no chance of recovery. She thinks that if Ben knew he had a chance of recovery by being placed on a ventilator, he would take it (10).

This case illustrates the point that, in making out an advance directive, an individual cannot envision all of the possible types of circumstances he might be in. Thus in writing an advance directive, one should not make instructions so specific or absolute as to preclude administration of medically beneficial treatment.

A complication in writing instructions for forgoing life-sustaining treatments is a legal trend to want "clear and convincing evidence" that a patient would not want the treatment in the particular situation in which he is found (12, 13). Again, an individual cannot envision all of the various circumstances he might be in medically when making out an advance directive, much less give detailed instructions for the various scenarios. A possible way of circumventing this problem is to include a statement in a durable power of attorney for health care document to the effect that, if one's wishes are not clear about using or forgoing a particular treatment in a particular circumstance, one wants one's designated proxy to use his or her judgment about what would be in one's best interests.

There are several problems health care providers may encounter in using advance directives. For one thing, patients may say they have these documents but forget to bring them to the health care facility or service so that they can be placed in the medical record and actually guide treatment decision making. Or again, it may not be understood that an advance directive is *not* the same thing as a Do-Not-Resuscitate Order, which must be written by a physician. Another common problem is that family members do not understand the legal status of the proxy decision maker named through a durable power of attorney for health care; namely, that this individual has the final decision regarding medical treatment and takes precedence over any (other) relative. This lack of understanding can result in family conflict. Or again, it may be unclear whether an individual still has the mental competency to make medical treatment decisions and, concomitantly, it will be unclear whether an advance directive should become operative.

The durable power of attorney for health care carries its own special problems. It is not unusual for an individual to ask a family member to serve as his proxy decision maker. However, it may be emotionally difficult for this family member to make a decision to "let go" of a loved one by forgoing life-sustaining treatments, even though this is what the individual in question would have wanted. In other words, acting as a proxy decision maker for medical treatments can prove a burdensome task to assume (11).

Further, residents of advanced age in long-term care facilities may have outlived the family members and friends who would be candidates for selection as their proxy decision maker. And if they have no one to designate to serve in this capacity, they are precluded from executing this type of advance directive (11).

Other Types of Advance Care Planning

Documents for advance care planning are not limited to those enacted by state legislation. One such document is the *Five Wishes* (14). This document includes not only the medical wishes but also the personal, emotional and spiritual wishes of seriously ill persons. Its five sections cover "The Person I Want to Make Care Decisions for Me When I Can't," "The Kind of Medical Treatment I Want or Don't Want," "How Comfortable I Want to Be," "How I Want People to Treat Me," and "What I Want My Loved Ones to Know."

Like the durable power of attorney for health care document, it allows one to designate a proxy decision maker. Like the living will, it allows one to give instructions regarding medical treatments at the very end of life. However, it goes beyond these two documents in offering choices about non-medical means of comfort care (e.g., being massaged with warm oils, having favorite music played, having religious readings and poems read aloud), about the environment in which one is to die (e.g., dying at home, having pictures of loved ones in one's room, having one's hand held and being talked to by others, having others by one's side praying), and about one's final communications to others (e.g., that one loves and forgives other people, how one wants to be remembered, one's desires for funeral services). The *Five Wishes* document is recognized as a legally valid advance directive in most states (14).

The Physician Orders for Life-Sustaining Treatment (POLST) Paradigm Initiative began in Oregon in 1991 under the auspices of the Center for Ethics in Health Care at Oregon Health & Science University (15). The project is now under the direction of the National POLST Paradigm Task Force (NPPTF) (16). This project has provided a model form which is being used in various states, with some modifications and refinements of the template (17). The POLST form (and its variants) translate a patient's values and wishes, whether expressed personally, by a proxy decision maker, or in an advance directive, into *actual medical orders* (18).

The process of executing a POLST form "starts with a conversation between health care professionals and patients" that "allows the patient to discuss his or her values, beliefs, and goals for care" while "the health care professional presents the patient's diagnosis, prognosis, and treatment alternatives" (19). They then reach "a shared decision about the patient's treatment plan" (19). The intent of the POLST form is to record the patient's treatment preferences as he or she nears the end of life (19). The POLST form can be used "to clarify whether the patient wants treatments provided to attempt to extend his/her life, wants to receive limited medical interventions or wants to let nature take its course and allow death to occur naturally" (19). Sections of the form address resuscitation, the use of medically assisted nutrition, and choices regarding comfort measures only versus various levels of medical interventions (18). A POLST form is portable across health care services—hospital, long-term care, home care, hospice, EMT services (18).

Not everyone is eligible to execute a POLST form. It is intended only for patients who are seriously ill or medically frail (17, 18). The rule of thumb is that POLST is intended for use by persons expected to die within 1 year (17).

Because POLST originated in the state of Oregon, some have wondered about the relationship between POLST and Oregon's "Death with Dignity" statute which allows what is called "physician assisted suicide" (PAS) or "physician aid-in-dying" (PAD) (see Chapter 11). The National POLST Paradigm

Task Force (NPPTF) has affirmed that the two "developed completely independently of each other by different groups with different goals" (19). The NPPTF has stated that "the National Physician Orders for Life-Sustaining Treatment Paradigm recognizes that allowing natural death to occur is not the same as providing a lethal prescription to intentionally cause death," and has affirmed that "neither the POLST Paradigm nor any POLST Form allows for PAS or PAD, nor does either authorize a health care professional to prescribe medication that would intentionally shorten life" (19).

CHAPTER SUMMARY

Key Terms and Concepts

principle of substituted judgment: a proxy decision maker attempts to reach the decision that the incapacitated person would make if he or she were able to choose, relying on written or oral directives explicitly given by the patient or on knowledge of the patient's beliefs, values, preferences, and life-long behavior patterns.

best interests standard: a proxy decision maker makes a choice that seeks to implement what is in the patient's best interests by reference to objective, societally shared criteria. It is sometimes expressed as choosing as a reasonable person in the patient's circumstances would.

advance directive: a legal document in which an individual makes provision for future medical treatment decisions in the event that he or she loses decision-making capacity.

living will: one type of advance directive in which an individual gives instructions to forgo life-sustaining treatments when he or she is suffering from a terminal illness (and death is expected in a short period of time) or in a state of permanent unconsciousness.

durable power of attorney for health care: one type of advance directive in which an individual legally designates someone as his or her proxy decision maker for times when he or she is incapacitated and cannot make treatment decisions.

Key Points

■ When a patient is not capable of making treatment decisions, a proxy decision maker acts on behalf of the patient. An individual may be legally designated as the proxy decision maker through a durable power of attorney for health care document, or as a court appointed guardian.

■ Whenever possible, a proxy decision maker should make treatment decisions on the basis of what the patient himself or herself would want done (*principle of substituted judgment*).

■ There are two types of legally recognized advance directives: the *living will* and the *durable power of attorney for health care*. These documents can be executed by mentally competent persons of legal age, but only for themselves.

■ The living will is *not* applicable to medical emergencies from which a patient can recover with appropriate treatment. It goes into effect only when the patient is suffering from a terminal illness (and death is expected in a short period of time) and the patient has lost the capacity to make his or her own treatment decisions. A living will may also apply to patients who are permanently unconscious.

■ A durable power of attorney for health care provides for a proxy decision maker who can assess the specific condition of the patient and engage in give-and-take discussion of medical alternatives. It is broader in scope than a living will, going into effect whenever a patient becomes incapacitated to make his or her own decisions, even temporarily.

■ At the present time the living will and durable power of attorney for health care documents are legally established by individual states. Generally, one can expect an advance directive executed in one state to be honored in other states.

■ The federal Patient Self-Determination Act requires all health care facilities and agencies to provide information about advance directives to patients, to inquire whether he or she has executed one, and to record the response on the patient's medical record. The law does *not* require anyone to execute an advance directive, but does require that health care facilities and agencies let people know that these documents are available if they wish to use them.

■ Advance directives are beneficial in promoting patient autonomy, protecting against the overuse of life-sustaining treatments, making health care providers more comfortable with complying with requests to forgo life-sustaining treatments, and helping to resolve conflicts about using or forgoing treatments without going to court.

■ Challenges in using advance directives include projecting what one would and would not want done in types of health situations one may never have experienced, and the fact that one cannot envision all the possible scenarios in which medical treatment decisions may have to be made. In giving treatment instructions, some room should be left for discretionary judgment.

■ There are documents for advance care planning in addition to those established by state legislation, such as the *Five Wishes* document and *POLST*.

FOR FURTHER DISCUSSION

1. Consider the case of Mel Langley at the beginning of the chapter. The physician Dr. Reynolds arranges a meeting to discuss the course of action to be taken.

   Role play this meeting. Participants should assume the roles of Dr. Reynolds, Mel's brother, Mel's two sisters, and radiation therapist Barbara O'Connor. The following points should be included in the conversation.

   - *Mel has executed a living will. Does it go into effect in his present condition?*
   - *Mel has executed a durable power of attorney for health care. Does it go into effect in his present condition?*
   - *Who should make the decision about using/forgoing medical treatments for Mel?*
   - *What principles should be used in arriving at a decision about using/forgoing medical treatments for Mel? And how do they apply to Mel's case?*
   - *Is there any other factual information that is needed to make a good decision?*

   After listening to this conversation, what do you think should be done about using/forgoing medical treatments for Mel?

2. Do an Internet search to obtain copies of the living will and durable power of attorney for health care from your home state. In small groups, review these documents. Do you have any questions about the content of these documents? About how to fill them out? Do you see any differences in the forms from different states? Are these differences significant?

3. Do you know anyone who has executed an advance directive? How did the person feel about doing this? Do you know of any cases in which an advance directive was used in making treatment decisions?

References

1. President's Commission for the Study of Ethical Problems in Medicine and Biomedical and Behavioral Research, *Deciding to Forego Life-Sustaining Treatment* (New York, NY: Concern for Dying, 1983; reprint).
2. Hastings Center, *Guidelines on the Termination of Life-Sustaining Treatment and the Care of the Dying* (Briarcliff Manor, NY: Hastings Center, 1987).
3. US Legal, "*Living Will Law & Legal Definition.*" http://definitions.uslegal.com/l/living-will. Accessed January 2016.

4. Patients Rights Council, "*Advance Directives: Definitions.*" http://www.patientsright-scouncil.org/site/advance-directives-definitions. Accessed January 2016.

5. Legalzoom, "*Living Will Glossary.*" https://www.legalzoom.com/knowl-edge/living-will/glossary/ living-will. Accessed January 2016.

6. Duhaime's Law Dictionary, "*Living Will Definition.*" http:// www.duhaime.org/LegalDictionary/L/LivingWill.aspx. Accessed January 2016.

7. The Free Dictionary—Legal Dictionary, "*Living Will.*" http://legal-dictionary.thefreedictionary.com/living+will. Accessed January 2016.

8. Commission on Legal Problems of the Elderly of the American Bar Association, "*10 Legal Myths About Advance Directives.*" http://ruralinstitute.umt.edu/transition/Handouts/10LegalMyths.pdf. Accessed January 2016.

9. Gregory E. Pence, *Medical Ethics Accounts of the Cases That Shaped and Define Medical Ethics*, 5th ed. (New York: McGraw-Hill, 2008).

10. Catholic Health Association of the United States, *The Patient Self-Determination Act* (St. Louis, MO: Catholic Health Association, 1991).

11. Nancy M.P. King, *Making Sense of Advance Directives*, rev. ed. (Washington, DC: Georgetown University Press, 1996).

12. George J. Annas, "Culture of Life' Politics at the Bedside The Case of Terri Schiavo," in *The Case of Terri Schiavo*, eds. Arthur Caplan, James J. McCartney, and Dominic A. Sisti (Amherst, NY: Prometheus Books, 2006).

13. Timothy E. Quill, "Terri Schiavo—A Tragedy Compounded," in *The Case of Terri Schiavo*, eds. Arthur Caplan, James J. McCartney, and Dominic A. Sisti (Amherst, NY: Prometheus Books, 2006).

14. Aging with Dignity, "*Five Wishes.*" https://agingwithdignity.org/ >Five Wishes > About Five Wishes > Preview. Accessed January 2016.

15. Center for Ethics in Health Care, Oregon Health & Science University, "*POLST.*" http://www.ohsu.edu/xd/education/continuing-education/center-for-ethics/ethics-programs/polst.cfm. Accessed January 2016.

16. National POLST, "*National POLST Paradigm Task Force.*" http://www.polst.org/about-the-national-polst-paradigm/national-task-force. Accessed January 2016.

17. National POLST, "*About the National POLST Paradigm.*" http://www.polst.org/about-the-national-polst-paradigm. Accessed January 2016.

18. Judy Citko, Alvin H. Moss, Margaret Carley, and Susan Tolle, *Fast Facts and Concepts #178 The National POLST Paradigm Initiative*, 2nd ed. (Sept. 2010). http://www.mcw.edu/FileLibrary/User/jrehm/fastfactpdfs/Concept178.pdf. Accessed January 2016.

19. National POLST Paradigm Task Force, "*Distinguishing POLST from Death with Dignity Statutes.*" (September 18, 2015). http://www.polst.org/wp-content/uploads/2015/11/2015.10.   05-DWD-POLST-Statement.pdf. Accessed January 2016.

Chapter 9

The Dilemma of Assisted Nutrition and Hydration

After an automobile accident at age 24, Nancy Cruzan was diagnosed as being in a vegetative state. She was apparently unconscious and unaware of her surroundings, unable to communicate, and unable to chew or swallow in a normal manner. After 4 years in this condition in a Missouri hospital, Nancy's family requested that the feeding tube that was keeping her alive be removed and that she be allowed to die. A court order, granting permission to withdraw the feeding tube, was overturned on appeal to the Missouri State Supreme Court. The question of removing Nancy's feeding tube eventually went to the U.S. Supreme Court (1). Both legally and ethically, the issue of withholding or withdrawing tube feeding has been so controversial that it deserves special attention among life-sustaining treatments.

What is known as *artificial nutrition and hydration* or *(medically) assisted nutrition and hydration* can take various forms. A needle may be inserted into a vein in the arm; this is known as *peripheral intravenous feeding*. Or a catheter may be inserted into a central vein near the heart, which is called *central intravenous feeding* or *total parenteral feeding* or *hyperalimentation*. Another form is the *nasogastric (NG) tube*, which consists of a thin plastic tube inserted through the nose into the stomach or into the first portion of the duodenum. A *gastrostomy tube* is inserted directly into the stomach, either surgically or through an incision made with the assistance of an endoscope (percutaneous endoscopic gastrostomy [PEG]). A *jejunostomy tube* is placed in the small intestine, either surgically or by a method similar to PEG tube placement (2, 3).

Assisted nutrition and hydration may be used on a short-term basis following surgery when the patient temporarily cannot eat (2). Such uses of assisted nutrition and hydration are not controversial. But assisted nutrition and hydration can also be used for longer periods of time in a variety of circumstances in which the patient cannot get adequate nutrition and hydration by normal means. A patient may be unable to swallow because of a stroke. Cancers can block the gastrointestinal tract. Enzymes necessary to absorb nutrients in the intestines may be inadequate. Or, while the patient may have a normal mouth, stomach, and intestinal tract, she may be adverse to or uninterested in eating (2). From an ethical point of view, assisted nutrition and hydration has been controversial when used for a prolonged period of time as a means (and sometimes the only means) of continuing to keep a patient alive.

In this chapter, you will learn about:

- The controversy surrounding whether assisted nutrition and hydration should be classified as "standard care" or as "medical treatment";
- The benefits and burdens of assisted nutrition and hydration;
- Common misunderstandings about assisted nutrition and hydration;
- Guidelines developed by the American Dietetic Association, the Alzheimer's Association, and the American Geriatrics Society for providing assisted nutrition and hydration.

Case Study

Barbara Ryan, a 70-year-old widow, is the kind of grandmother whose life revolves around her grandchildren. She is constantly doing things with them and taking them places. Barbara has always enjoyed reasonably good health. Everyone is surprised when she collapses at a church picnic to which she has taken three of her grandchildren.

At the hospital, Barbara's daughter Ann and son Robert are told that Barbara has suffered a stroke. Because of this, she cannot swallow normally. Ann and Robert have no qualms about consenting to the placement of the feeding tube for their mother.

After a week, Barbara is transferred to the Forest Glen Nursing Home. Her family visits her frequently. Because Barbara's grandchildren are anxious for her to get well, Barbara's daughter and son insist that her physician and the nursing home staff do everything necessary for her recovery.

However, Barbara eventually lapses into a semiconscious state. She doesn't recognize family members or friends when they come to visit her. She is bedridden, listless, and suffers periodic bouts of aspiration pneumonia caused by the feeding tube.

After their mother has been in this condition for 2 years, Ann and Robert begin to reassess their directive to the physician and nursing home staff to "do everything" for their mother. They recall a statement she made while taking care of their dying father. She said most emphatically that she was "ready to die when God wanted to take her" and wanted "no heroic measures to interfere with God's plan."

Ann goes to court to be named her mother's legal guardian. With the agreement of her brother, Ann requests that the tube feeding that is keeping their mother alive be stopped. Barbara's physician agrees to this request.

However, the facility's dietitian, Ron Kennedy, who has been involved in Barbara's care for the past 2 years, becomes very upset when he hears that Barbara's feeding tube will be removed. He believes it is wrong to deny any person food and water. In fact, Ron tells the facility's administrator that, if Barbara's feeding tube is removed, he will have to consider quitting his job because he does not want to be part of a resident being "starved to death."

■ ■ ■

"Standard Care" or "Medical Treatment"?

The dietitian in our case believes that it is wrong to deny any person food and water. One issue that arose early in the debate about assisted nutrition and hydration is whether it should be classified as "standard nursing care" and hence should always be provided, or whether it should be regarded as a "medical treatment" to be used or forgone on the same basis as other life-sustaining treatments.

Those who regard assisted nutrition and hydration as standard nursing care have put forward several arguments in support of their view. They point out that, while medical treatment is therapeutic, nutrition and hydration are not because they will not cure a disease (4, 5). However, it could be said in rebuttal that not all recognized medical treatments cure disease. For example, kidney dialysis does not cure the problem of kidney failure, but simply provides a way of circumventing the problem. Similarly, assisted nutrition and hydration circumvents problems with eating.

It has also been argued that withholding or withdrawing food and fluids is different than withholding or withdrawing medical therapies because of its finality. Withholding or withdrawing food and fluids ensures death, whereas in the case of removing a patient from a ventilator, for example, the patient may surprise us and breathe on her own (4–7). However, this line of argument ignores the fact that stopping dialysis inevitably results in a patient's death, as does a decision not to perform cardiopulmonary resuscitation when a cardiac arrest occurs (8). Moreover, in the case of an unconscious patient, a ventilator and assisted nutrition and hydration are alike in that both replace normal bodily functions that are compromised by that patient's illness (9).

Some assisted feeding devices are surgically inserted, and this is certainly a medical procedure. In addition, assisted nutrition and hydration is used by a physician's order, and are monitored by a physician or someone working under a physician's direction (9).

In the case of Nancy Cruzan, the U.S. Supreme Court took the position that her feeding tube was a "medical procedure" (10). Similarly, the American Dietetic Association has taken the position that assisted nutrition and hydration is to be considered a "medical intervention" (11). On this view, using or forgoing assisted nutrition and hydration is decided on the same basis as using or forgoing other medical life-sustaining procedures, viz., considering the benefits and burdens of the procedure and the wishes of the patient (see Chapter 7).

In 2004, the question of the status of assisted nutrition and hydration was resurrected by an address given by Pope John Paul II to a conference on vegetative state patients (see Chapter 10) held at the Vatican. John Paul II stated the view that "the administration of water and food, even when provided by artificial means, always represents a natural means of preserving life, not a medical act" (12). A subsequent clarification of this papal address from the Vatican Congregation for the Doctrine of the Faith reaffirmed this view but indicated that assisted nutrition and hydration may be forgone for a patient if this procedure is not effective in providing the patient with nourishment or if the procedure proves excessively burdensome for the patient or causes significant physical discomfort (13). This is not a contradictory position because, within

Catholic moral theology, early discussions of "extraordinary," nonobligatory treatments "did not necessarily concern medical acts per se, but also included actions like moving one's residence to a more suitable climate and the use of 'delicate' foods" (14; see also 15).

Yet another position on the status of assisted nutrition and hydration is that it is a combination of both medical treatment and basic health care: the method by which nutrition and hydration is delivered is a medical procedure but the material conveyed (food and water) belongs to the category of basic health care (15). Otherwise stated:

> In itself, the provision of food and water (by whatever means) is the ordinary way of sustaining a patient's life and a minimal part of the care we owe to others. . . . While the act of feeding a person is not itself a medical act, the insertion of a tube, monitoring of the tube and patient, and prescription of the substances to be provided, do involve a degree of medical and/or nursing expertise. To insert a feeding tube is a medical decision subject to the normal criteria for medical intervention. (16)

This position likewise admits the permissibility of forgoing assisted nutrition and hydration if it proves futile or excessively burdensome (15, 16).

A common denominator in the categorization of assisted nutrition and hydration as a medical treatment, in the position of the Vatican, and in the position that assisted nutrition and hydration is a combination of medical treatment and basic health care, is a recognition that it is legitimate to forgo this procedure in some cases and that this may be determined using the principle of weighing benefits and burdens.

The Benefits and Burdens of Assisted Nutrition and Hydration

Assisted nutrition and hydration can have distinct benefits for some patients. It offers the very fundamental benefit of "prolonging life in patients who are unable to take adequate nutrition by mouth" (17). It can also benefit patients by providing time to treat underlying medical problems or to clarify the patient's prognosis (17). Assisted nutrition and hydration may help to stabilize a patient's physical status following severe trauma (18). It may allow a restful healing time for a diseased or damaged gastrointestinal tract, or serve as a means to provide nutrition and hydration during a restoration period following surgery (18). It can serve to reverse malnutrition and dehydration (18).

Cheryl Arenella, MD, MPH, who has extensive experience in the field of Hospice and palliative care, offers the following examples of situations in which assisted nutrition and hydration are helpful to patients who are seriously ill:

- A person who has a mechanical blockage of his or her mouth, esophagus, or stomach, but is otherwise functioning fairly well, especially if this person is experiencing hunger, is likely to benefit if a tube is placed below the blockage in order to be able to receive nutrition and fluids. This is the case in many persons who suffer from head and neck or esophageal cancer, especially in the earlier stages of the cancer.
- In some cases, when a blocked bowel develops, such as in the spread of ovarian cancer, but the person is otherwise fairly functional, total parental nutrition (TPN) has been helpful in allowing that person to live and function longer than without the treatment.
- A person who has a temporary bout of severe nausea and vomiting or has diarrhea causing serious dehydration can often benefit from a short course of intravenous fluids to rest the bowel.
- Some persons with cachexia (a condition where the person keeps losing weight and does not eat well) due to HIV disease appear to benefit from assisted nutrition and hydration, especially those who have no active infection at the time of receiving it (19).

On the other hand, there are cases in which assisted nutrition and hydration simply will not work and be effective in prolonging life. For example, a patient may be suffering from such severe heart, kidney, or liver failure that his body cannot process, metabolize, or excrete the nutrients or fluids supplied through the feeding device (3). Or again, it may be virtually impossible to attach a feeding tube to a patient with nearly total body burn (20). A feeding tube may not work because the tube itself has developed complications such as infection or bleeding, or because it has become entangled in the bowels so that the bowel tissue dies and can no longer absorb nutrients (21). In such cases, assisted nutrition and hydration is a futile procedure in a very basic physiological sense (see Chapter 7) and, according to the principle of weighing benefits and burdens, there is no moral obligation to use it.

Assisted nutrition and hydration also carries burdens of physical risks and complications. These have been enumerated by Dr. Cheryl Arenella:

- TPN (total parental nutrition) and central catheters can cause infection at the site of the catheter and in the catheter itself as well as sepsis (a generalized life-threatening infection). Pneumothorax (collapse of the lung) can occur at the time of inserting the catheter. Thrombosis (clots in the vein) can occur, causing local swelling. Sometimes these clots can travel to other parts of the body such as the brain or lung and can be life-threatening. Cardiac arrhythmias (irregularities of the heart beat) as well as electrolyte disturbances such as low sodium, low potassium, or low blood sugar can occur. These are all potentially life-threatening.

- A nasogastric tube can cause choking and extreme discomfort at placement and afterwards. At the time of insertion, it can be misplaced in the trachea and cause pneumonia. The tube can cause erosions and abrasions, even perforations (holes) in the nasal passages, esophagus and stomach, and can cause acute and chronic bleeding. Aspiration pneumonia is a risk whenever an NG tube is in place. If a person is confused, he or she may need restraints to keep him or her from pulling the tube out. This can cause a whole host of problems, including psychic distress and increased agitation and anxiety, skin breakdown due to immobility, pneumonia due to immobility, and injury from restraints . . .

- A gastrostomy tube requires anesthesia during placement and has risks associated with the use of anesthesia. There is also a risk of infection of the abdominal wall and peritonitis (life-threatening infection of the abdominal cavity). Gastrointestinal bleeding, blockage of the bowel or perforation of the bowel may occur. Diarrhea from the feeding formula is fairly common. Aspiration pneumonia is also common. If the person requires restraints to keep from pulling the tube out, the same complications listed above can occur.

- Intravenous fluids require IV tubing, with associated pain on insertion. Localized infection or cellulitis (a more serious infection of the skin that can spread) can occur. Thrombophlebitis (clotting in the vein) can occur and cause swelling and discomfort. Fluid overload is possible, causing swelling of the legs, arms, and body. Electrolyte imbalances such as low sodium or low potassium are common (19).

In sum, assisted nutrition and hydration is a mixed blessing. While it can benefit a patient, there are also definite burdens which can be associated with it. As with all treatments, decisions about using or forgoing assisted nutrition and hydration must be made on a case-by-case basis by considering the benefits and burdens of this procedure for a particular patient.

Common Misunderstandings About Assisted Nutrition and Hydration

The dietitian in our case study describes the removal of the feeding tube from Mrs. Ryan as "starving a patient to death." We often hear this phrase used in cases where a decision is made to withhold or withdraw assisted nutrition and hydration. But this description involves some misconceptions about forgoing assisted nutrition and hydration.

First, the phrase "starving a patient to death" carries the connotation that we are doing something to cause the patient's death, or engaging in an act of euthanasia. Second, the description "starving a patient to death" conjures up images of a painful, agonizing death.

One definition of euthanasia is "an action or an omission which of itself or by intention causes death, in order that all suffering may in this way be eliminated" (22). If we are dealing with some underlying fatal pathology which makes the assisted nutrition and hydration necessary in the first place (e.g., a stroke which makes the patient unable to swallow), the removal or withholding of the feeding device merely allows that fatal pathology to take its natural course. It is the underlying fatal pathology, not the absence of assisted nutrition and hydration, that is the direct cause of death. Further, the intent behind the removal or withdrawal of assisted nutrition and hydration is important. If the purpose is one of intentionally ending the patient's life before death occurs naturally, then we are dealing with a case of euthanasia. On the other hand, if the purpose is to relieve the patient of a procedure that is of limited usefulness or unreasonably burdensome, then this decision can be seen as different than a decision to kill a patient (18, 23). Thus withholding or withdrawing assisted nutrition and hydration under these conditions, namely, when an underlying fatal pathology directly causes death and the intent is to relieve the patient of a non-beneficial or very burdensome treatment, does not constitute an act of euthanasia on our part.

Second, the description "starving a patient to death" conjures up images of a painful, agonizing death. It is simply not true that a patient who is not given assisted nutrition and hydration will die in this way. For one thing, sensations of hunger and thirst can be relieved without using assisted nutrition and hydration. For example, ice chips or glycerin swabbing of the mouth can be used to relieve the thirst of dehydrated patients (24, 25). Further, studies involving assisted nutrition and hydration for patients with varying degrees of consciousness have indicated that withdrawal of the feeding device does not cause suffering associated with hunger and dehydration (14). Moreover, there is evidence that patients who are allowed to die without assisted nutrition and hydration may die more comfortably than patients who receive conventional amounts of intravenous hydration (26). Dehydration can reduce swelling and increase comfort in a patient suffering from edema (swelling of the body caused by excess body fluids) or ascites (fluid in the abdominal cavity). Cough and congestion may be lessened because secretions in the lungs are diminished. A dehydrated person has less urine output so that problems with incontinence are lessened. Since there is less fluid in the gastrointestinal tract with dehydration, a patient may experience a decrease in nausea, vomiting, bloating, and regurgitation. Indeed, dehydration leads to death in ways that produce a sedative effect on the brain just before death, thus decreasing the need for pain medication (19, 11, 25, 26). Consider the following actual case:

> David was a 64-year-old man with recurrent metastatic cancer of the larynx and tongue. Before being referred to the hospice program, he had received several years of therapy including surgery, radiation, and chemotherapy. He had massive facial and neck deformity with superimposed edema, which had resulted from treatment and recurrent disease. He had a continuous flow of secretions from the mouth and the tracheostomy site. His severe pain was managed with morphine sulfate, but maintaining his airway was a serious challenge. Although secretions could be removed by suctioning, the growing tumor and increasing edema threatened total airway occlusion.
>
> The patient, who was alert and oriented and had been feeding himself through a gastric tube, then decided to discontinue tube feedings. He lived 27 days after this decision. During that time, his appearance and comfort improved remarkably. Family members noted that the lessening facial edema made him look more like his usual self. The decrease in the neck edema resulted in a patent airway, which consequently eased the patient's breathing. A decrease in oral secretions also greatly added to his comfort. David remained mentally alert and interacted with his family. His pain was managed with approximately half of the morphine doses previously necessary. His death came quietly and comfortably. (27)

Providing food and water to a patient has been seen by some as a symbol of care and concern for that person. For this reason, they believe that tube feedings should always be provided to those who need it physically. But nutrition and hydration supplied by medical means is not always a good expression of loving care and concern:

> Food and water are certainly significant symbols, but the social experience associated with the giving and receiving of food and water may be

equally important. The patient receiving intravenous fluids, lying alone in a hospital bed, is having a much less rewarding experience than the patient in a personalized room being given ice chips by a concerned caregiver. Both are receiving water, but there are few other similarities. (28)

Finally, what are the social and psychological effects of feeding techniques? With tube feedings, the caregiver may focus more attention on technical aspects, such as positioning the tube and checking the gastric residual, than on the patient. If feeding proceeds smoothly, contact between the patient and caregiver can be minimal. Moreover, the patient has no control over tube feedings except to pull out the tube. In contrast, during hand feedings the caregiver may be more attentive and affectionate, talking with the patient or holding his or her hand. Patients with few other ways of exercising control can still determine the timing, pace, and content of hand feeding. . . . Hand feedings that provide inadequate nutrition may meet more of the patient's needs than tube feedings that deliver adequate calories impersonally. The psychosocial effects of feeding techniques are especially important when the goal is supportive care. (29)

In sum, we must keep in mind that medical technologies can never replace personal presence and the human touch in caregiving.

For further discussion of assisted nutrition and hydration in the case of patients with disorders of consciousness, see Chapter 10.

Professional Association Guidelines

In working through difficult ethical dilemmas, health care workers can be assisted by guidelines developed by professional associations. In 1987 the American Dietetic Association published a position paper *Issues in Feeding the Terminally Ill Adult* (25). According to this position paper, it is legitimate to forgo assisted nutrition and hydration in such cases when some or all of the following conditions are present:

- Death is imminent, within hours or a few days.
- Tube feeding will probably worsen the condition, symptoms, or pain, such as during shock, when pulmonary edema, vomiting, or aspiration would cause further complications.
- A competent patient has expressed an informed preference not to receive aggressive nutrition support which would be ineffective in improving the

quality of life and/or which may be perceived by the patient as undignified, degrading, and physically or emotionally unacceptable.

■ If available and legally recognized, written directives such as the "living will" or "durable power of attorney for medical care" may indicate the preference of an incompetent patient. Otherwise, the next of kin or guardian of an incompetent patient should be consulted about the patient's probable preference for the level of nutrition intervention (25).

These guidelines are consistent with the ethical principles we have been using for making decisions about life-sustaining treatments (see Chapter 7). The first and second bullet points fit with the principle of weighing benefits and burdens. The first bullet point can be interpreted as an application of the category of futile treatment, and the second bullet point deals with burdens which can be imposed on a patient by assisted nutrition and hydration. The third and fourth bullet points embody the concept of patient autonomy.

The American Dietetic Association subsequently published another position paper *Ethical and Legal Issues in Nutrition, Hydration, and Feeding* in 2008. (11) A section of this paper entitled "Suggested ethical deliberations about nutrition and hydration" contains the following points relevant to assisted nutrition and hydration:

1. The patient's expressed desire for extent of medical care is a primary guide for determining the level of nutrition intervention . . .
2. The expected benefits, in contrast to the potential burdens, of nonoral feeding must be evaluated by the health care team and discussed with the patient. The focus of care should include the patient's physical and psychological comfort . . .
3. Consider whether or not nutrition, either oral or artificial, will improve the patient's quality of life during the final stages of life.
4. Consider whether or not nutrient support, either oral or artificial, can be expected to provide the patient with emotional comfort, decreased anxiety about disease cachexia, improved self-esteem with cosmetic benefits, improved interpersonal relationships, or relief from fear of abandonment.
5. If death is imminent and feeding will not alter condition consider whether or not nutrient support will be burdensome . . .
6. When tube feeding or parenteral feeding is being considered:
   a. The patient's informed preference for the level of nutritional intervention is primary. The patient or substitute decision maker should be advised on how to accomplish whatever feeding the patient desires.

b. When palliative care is the agreed goal nutritional support must be part of the palliative plan. A palliative care plan does not automatically preclude aggressive nutrition support. The decision to forgo "heroic" medical treatment does not preclude baseline nutrition support. All options for nutritional support can be considered.

c. Feeding may not be desirable if death is expected within hours or a few days and the effects of partial dehydration or the withdrawal of nutrition support will not adversely alter patient comfort . . .

d. The potential benefits versus burdens of tube feeding or parenteral feeding should be weighed on the basis of specific facts concerning the patient's medical and mental status, as well as on the facility's options and limitations.

e. Facility options and limitations—One should consider the following:

(1) Lack of staffing—no one to manage or monitor feeding

(2) Too costly without financial help

(3) If a feeding strategy is started on one site it will have to be stopped when the patient is transferred to another site, which can lead to a sense of abandonment (11).

The position paper *Ethical and Legal Issues in Nutrition, Hydration, and Feeding* "affirms the patient's right to self-determination as the overriding principle" (11). This emphasis on patient autonomy is embodied in points 1 and 9a. However, the principle of weighing benefits and burdens is also invoked in points 3, 7, and 9f. In fact, points 6 and 9g can be interpreted as describing types of benefits and burdens to be taken into account.

This position paper similarly recognizes the role of an ethics committee in health care facilities. In recommending that "facilities should provide and distribute written protocols for the provision of and termination of tube feedings and parenteral feedings," it is mentioned that "the institution's ethics committee, if available, should assist in establishing and implementing defined, written guidelines for nutrition support protocol" (11). Or again, if a physician writes a diet order that the facility's registered dietitian does not agree with, "appeal to the facility's ethics mechanism (committee or consultant)" is advised (11). Moreover, this position paper affirms that "registered dietitians should serve as active members of institutional ethics committees" (11). Registered dietitians will bring to ethical discussions the technical knowledge of how to achieve desired feeding goals (11), and they "often have specific knowledge regarding the individual patient's preference because they discuss feeding issues with the patient and family" (11).

Persons with advanced dementia generally experience eating difficulties (30). Thus the question arises of continuing hand feeding or providing medically assisted nutrition and hydration for them (30).

The position paper *Assisted Oral Feeding and Tube Feeding* issued by the Alzheimer's Association in 2011 contends that "in comparison with assisted oral feeding, long-term tube feeding offers no advantages and incurs a number of disadvantages" for persons with advanced Alzheimer's disease (31). Specifically, research on tube feeding indicates that it does not usually improve the nutritional status of such patients, prevent or lower the incidence of aspiration pneumonia, or reduce skin breakdown or the likelihood of pressure sores (31). Very importantly, "there is no average difference in longevity between persons with advanced Alzheimer's disease who are tube fed and those provided with assistance in oral feeding" (31). Among the disadvantages of tube feeding are an increased risk of diarrhea (31), increased use of physical restrains to prevent patients from pulling out the feeding tube (31), and denying the patient "the gratifications of tasting preferred foods and the emotional and relational benefits of interacting with a caregiver through assisted oral feeding" (31). Thus the Alzheimer's Association takes the position that "it is ethically permissible to withhold nutrition and hydration artificially administered by vein or gastric tube when the person with Alzheimer's disease or dementia is in the end stages of the disease and is no longer able to receive food or water by mouth" (31). The rationale for this ethical judgment clearly involves the principle of weighing benefits and burdens of treatment. This does not mean, however, that such patients are simply abandoned. The position paper goes on to affirm that "assisted oral feeding should be available to all persons with advanced Alzheimer's disease" (31), that neglect in this area should not be tolerated (31), and that efforts should be made to educate caregivers in techniques of assisted oral feeding (31).

The same conclusion was reached by the American Geriatrics Society in their *Feeding Tubes in Advanced Dementia Position Statement* of 2013: "the benefits versus the burdens of tube feeding do not support its use in older adults with advanced dementia" (31). This position paper likewise reports that tube feeding has not been shown to prevent aspiration, heal pressure wounds, improve nutritional status, or decrease mortality in patients with advanced dementia (30). It does not have these benefits for persons with advanced dementia. Moreover, the position paper reports that tube feeding may be accompanied by substantial burdens including recurrent or new onset aspiration, tube-associated and aspiration-related infection, increased oral secretions that are difficult to manage, discomfort, tube malfunction, and pressure wounds (30). Persons suffering from advanced dementia may need to be restrained, physically or chemically, to prevent them from pulling out the feeding tube (30). In fact, studies have shown that long-term care residents with advanced dementia and a feeding tube frequently need to be taken to a hospital emergency room to address tube-related complications (30). In sum, the report recommends that, rather than resorting to tube feeding for patients with advanced dementia, careful hand-feeding should be offered (30).

CHAPTER SUMMARY

Key Terms and Concepts

principle of patient autonomy: self-determination; an individual's right to hold views, make choices, and take actions based on personal values and beliefs.

principle of weighing benefits and burdens: A life-sustaining treatment ought to be used if it provides more benefits than burdens. It is morally permissible to forgo (i.e., withhold or withdraw) a life-sustaining treatment if the burdens of the treatment outweigh its benefits or if the treatment is useless or futile.

Key Points

- The use of assisted nutrition and hydration on a short-term basis is not controversial. From an ethical point of view, what has been debated is the use of assisted nutrition and hydration for a prolonged period of time as a means (and sometimes the only means) of keeping a patient alive.
- Assisted nutrition and hydration has been variously categorized as standard nursing care; as medical treatment; as a natural, nonmedical means of preserving life; and as a hybrid of medical treatment and basic health care.
- Procedures for providing assisted nutrition and hydration have burdens as well as benefits attached to them.
- Forgoing assisted nutrition and hydration in the presence of an underlying fatal pathology which directly causes death and with the intent of relieving the patient of a procedure that is of limited benefit or unreasonably burdensome, does not constitute an act of euthanasia.
- Comfort care can be provided to patients apart from using assisted nutrition and hydration. In fact, patients may die more comfortably without assisted nutrition and hydration than with it.
- Professional associations, such as the American Dietetic Association, the Alzheimer's Association, and the American Geriatrics Society, have provided guidelines to assist in making decisions about using or forgoing assisted nutrition and hydration.

FOR FURTHER DISCUSSION

1. Consider the case of Barbara Ryan at the beginning of this chapter. Since dietitian Ron Kennedy disagrees with the decision to withdraw the

feeding tube from Barbara, he should, according to the American Dietetic Association, take his concerns to the ethics committee of the Forest Glen Nursing Home.

Role play this ethics consult. You will need participants to represent Barbara Ryan's daughter Ann, Barbara's son Robert, dietitian Ron Kennedy, and members of the ethics committee.

- *What considerations is Ann likely to bring forward in support of removing the feeding tube from her mother? Do these arguments hold up?*
- *What is the dietitian Ron Kennedy likely to think and feel? What considerations might he raise against withdrawing the feeding tube? Do these arguments hold up?*
- *What ethical principles should be brought forward by members of the ethics committee? And how do these principles apply to Barbara's case?*
- *What ethical guidelines from the American Dietetic Association are relevant to this case?*
- *After listening to each point of view and considering the relevant ethical principles and guidelines, can the group reach agreement on what should be done in the case of Barbara Ryan?*

2. Stephen Marshall, 67, has been fighting colon cancer for 5 years. He has undergone numerous rounds of chemotherapy. Initially, the chemotherapy seemed to stop the growth of the cancer, but in the last 5 months it has been ineffective. For this reason, Stephen decides to discontinue the treatments.

   Stephen's condition continues to deteriorate. Because he has become so debilitated and the caregiving demands on his wife have become so great, he is admitted to Mercy Care Center under its hospice program. Because of the cancerous growth blocking his intestinal tract, Stephen cannot get much nutrition by normal means. In consultation with his oncologist, Stephen decides against having a feeding tube placed. Stephen tells everyone that he is "ready to die" and just wants to be kept as comfortable as possible until that time comes. Ten days later, Stephen dies.

   A few days later two certified nursing assistants (CNAs) who had cared for Stephen go to the facility's director of nursing (DON) to express concern that a feeding tube had not been used for Stephen. Alice and Diane say that they can understand withholding a feeding tube from a dying resident who is mentally "out of it" and doesn't know what is going on, but they can't deal with withholding feeding from a resident who is mentally alert and talks to them when they come into the room—even though they know the resident is near death and doesn't say that he is hungry. The DON suggests that Alice and Diane meet with Mercy's Ethics Committee to discuss their concerns.

Suppose you are a member of Mercy's Ethics Committee.

- *What would you say to the CNAs Alice and Diane?*
- *What factual information about tube feeding for persons who are imminently dying is relevant?*
- *How does this factual information connect with relevant ethical principles?*

You might want to role play the conversation with Alice and Diane.

References

1. Gregory E. Pence, *Classic Cases in Medical Ethics*, 2nd ed. (New York: McGraw-Hill, 1995), Chap. 1.
2. David Major, MD, "The Medical Procedures for Providing Food and Water: Indications and Effects" in *By No Extraordinary Means: The Choice to Forgo Life-Sustaining Food and Water*, ed. Joanne Lynn (Bloomington, IN: Indiana University Press, 1986).
3. Myles Sheehan, S.J., "Feeding Tubes: Sorting Out the Issues," *Health Progress* 82/6 (November–December 2001): 22–27.
4. Gilbert Meilaender, "On Removing Food and Water: Against the Stream," *Hastings Center Report* 14/6 (December 1984): 11–13.
5. New Jersey State Catholic Conference, "Providing Food and Fluids to Severely Brain Damaged Patients," *Origins* 16/32 (January 22, 1987): 582–84.
6. Patrick G. Derr, "Nutrition and Hydration as Elective Therapy: Brophy and Jobes from an Ethical and Historical Perspective," *Issues in Law & Medicine* 2/1 (1986): 25–38.
7. Patrick G. Derr, "Why Food and Fluids Can Never Be Denied," *Hastings Center Report* 16/1 (February 1986): 28–30.
8. Dennis Brodeur, "Is a Decision to Forgo Tube Feeding for Another a Decision to Kill?," *Issues in Law and Medicine* 6/4 (1991): 395–406.
9. American Academy of Neurology, "Position of the American Academy of Neurology on Certain Aspects of the Care and Management of the Persistent Vegetative State Patient," *Neurology* 39 (January 1989): 125–26, reprinted in James J. Walter and Thomas A. Shannon (eds.), *Quality of Life: The New Medical Dilemma* (New York: Paulist Press, 1990).
10. Cruzan v. Director, *Missouri Department of Health*, 110 S. Ct. 2841 (1990).

11. American Dietetic Association, "Position of the American Dietetic Association: Ethical and Legal Issues in Nutrition, Hydration, and Feeding," *Journal of the American Dietetic Association* 108 (2008): 873–82.

12. John Paul II, "Care for Patients in a 'Permanent' Vegetative State," *Origins* 33/43 (April 8, 2004): 737–40.

13. Congregation for the Doctrine of the Faith, Commentary on *Responses to Certain Questions of the United States Conference of Catholic Bishops Concerning Artificial Nutrition and Hydration* (August 1, 2007). https://www.etwn.com/library/CURIA/cdfaliment.htm. Accessed January 2016. See also United States Conference of Catholic Bishops, *Ethical and Religious Directives for Catholic Health Care Services*, 5th ed., no. 58, http://www.usccb.org. Accessed January 2016.

14. Dan O'Brien, John Paul Slosar, and Anthony R. Tersigni, "Utilitarian Pessimism, Human Dignity, and the Vegetative State A Practical Analysis of the Papal Allocution," *The National Catholic Bioethics Quarterly* 4/3 (Autumn 2004): 497–512.

15. Kevin D. O'Rourke, O.P., "The Catholic Tradition on Forgoing Life Support," *The National Catholic Bioethics Quarterly* 5/3 (Autumn 2005): 537–53.

16. Bishops Committee on Doctrine and Morals (Australian Catholic Bishops' Conference), Bishops Committee for Health Care (Australia), and Catholic Health Australia, "*Briefing Note on the Obligation to Provide Nutrition and Hydration*" (September 3, 2004). https://www.catholic.org.au/commission-documents/bishops-commission-for-doctrine-and-morals-1/438-briefing-note-on-the-obligation-to-provide-nutrition-and-hydration-1/file. Accessed January 2016.

17. Bernard Lo and Laurie Dornbrand, "Understanding the Benefits and Burdens of Tube Feedings," *Archives of Internal Medicine* 149/9 (September 1989): 1925–26.

18. Pikes Peak Forum for Health Care, "*Decisions About the End of Life . . . Help for Those Who Must Decide.*" (March 2008). http://www.pikespeakforum.org/PDF/PPFHCbookletMar2008.pdf. Accessed January 2016.

19. Cheryl Arenella, "*Artificial Nutrition and Hydration: Beneficial or Harmful?*" (2005). http://www.americanhospice.org/index.php?option=com_content&task=view&id=48&Itemid=8. Accessed January 2009.

20. Joanne Lynn and James F. Childress, "Must Patients Always Be Given Food and Water?" in *By No Extraordinary Means: The Choice to Forgo Life-Sustaining Food and Water*, ed. Joanne Lynn (Bloomington, IN: Indiana University Press, 1986).

21. Daniel P. Sulmasy, "Preserving Life? The Vatican & PVS," *Commonweal* 134/21 (December 7, 2007): 16–18.

22. Congregation for the Doctrine of the Faith, *Declaration on Euthanasia* (Washington, DC: United States Catholic Conference, 1980).

23. Committee for Pro-Life Activities of the National Conference of Catholic Bishops, "Nutrition and Hydration: Moral and Pastoral Reflections," *Origins* 21/44 (April 9, 1992): 705-12.

24. Hastings Center, *Guidelines on the Termination of Life-Sustaining Treatment and the Care of the Dying* (Briarcliff Manor, NY: Hastings Center, 1987).

25. American Dietetic Association, "Position of the American Dietetic Association: Issues in Feeding the Terminally Ill Adult," *American Dietetic Association Journal*, 87 (January-April 1987): 78-85.

26. Joyce C. Zerwekh, "The Dehydration Question," *Nursing* 83 (January 1983): 47–51.

27. Shirley Ann Smith, "Controversies in Hydrating the Terminally Ill Patient," *Journal of Intravenous Nursing* 20/4 (July/August 1997): 193–200.

28. Phyllis Schmitz and Merry O'Brien, "Observations on Nutrition and Hydration in Dying Cancer Patients" in *By No Extraordinary Means: The Choice to Forgo Life-Sustaining Food and Water*, ed. Joanne Lynn (Bloomington, IN: Indiana University Press, 1986).

29. Bernard Lo and Laurie Dornbrand, "Guiding the Hand That Feeds: Caring for the Demented Elderly," *New England Journal of Medicine* 311/6 (August 9, 1984): 402–4.

30. American Geriatrics Society, *Feeding Tubes in Advanced Dementia Position Statement.* (May 2013). http://www.americangeriatrics.org/files/documents/feeding.tubes.advanced.dementia.pdf. Accessed January 2016.

31. Alzheimer's Association, *Assisted Oral Feeding and Tube Feeding.* http://www.alz.org/documents_custom/statements/Assisted_Oral_Tube_Feeding.pdf. Accessed January 2016.

Chapter 10

Treatment Decisions for Vegetative State Patients

Three highly publicized court cases concerning the withdrawal of life-sustaining treatments have involved young adult women: Karen Ann Quinlan, Nancy Cruzan, and Terri Schiavo. In the case of Karen Ann Quinlan, at issue was the removal of a ventilator. In the cases of Nancy Cruzan and Terri Schiavo, the removal of a feeding tube proved controversial. What these women shared in common was the diagnosis of a disorder of consciousness known as a permanent vegetative state (1).

In this chapter, you will learn:

- The conventional medical view of the vegetative state;
- Recent medical advances in studying and treating patients in this condition;

- The particular set of ethical issues which arise in making decisions about life-sustaining treatments for these patients;
- How the ethical principles of autonomy, weighing benefits and burdens, and substituted judgment apply to these treatment decisions.

Case Study

Lucas Duarte, 35, and Carla Munoz, 32, have been married for 6 years. They have two children, Daniela, 4, and Christopher, 2. Both Lucas and Carla have established careers as attorneys.

Late one afternoon, as she is on her way to pick up her children at the day-care center, Carla's car is hit broadside by a pick-up truck which has run a stop sign. She is unconscious when the paramedics arrive and take her to the hospital emergency room.

When Lucas arrives at the hospital, he is told that Carla has suffered severe head trauma. She is in the intensive care unit (ICU) and has been placed on a ventilator.

Three weeks go by, and Carla remains "out of it." There are periods of time when her eyes are open but she doesn't seem aware of anyone in the room. She doesn't speak, and when the doctor tries to get her to respond to simple commands, she doesn't. She is now able to be taken off the ventilator and can breathe on her own, but she must be fed through a tube. A neurologist who examines Carla diagnoses her as being in a "vegetative state."

Carla is transferred to the Woodlands Care Center. Her care at the nursing home includes tube feeding, maintaining skin care and appropriate hygiene, range of motion exercises to minimize limb contracture, and time sitting out of bed.

A month after admission to the Woodlands Care Center—and 7 weeks after the accident that put her in this condition—Carla develops pneumonia. She is again examined by a neurologist, who tells Lucas that his wife is now in a "persistent vegetative state" and that he will have to make decisions about the kinds of treatments which should and should not be provided for his wife.

Without hesitation, Lucas insists that antibiotics—and any other treatment medically indicated—be provided for his wife. It is too soon, he believes, to give up on the possibility of his wife's recovery. He himself has seen several cases of patients who were written off as "hopeless" by doctors but who eventually recovered. Besides, he points out that his wife is still young, only

32 years old—much too young to be allowed to die. Indeed, for the sake of their two young children who need a mother, Lucas wants "everything possible" done to save Carla.

John Miller is the physical therapist supervising Carla's range of motion exercises. He personally is glad that Carla's husband has made this decision. After all, how could health care professionals let someone die whose eyes are open?

■ ■ ■

Disorders of Consciousness

Consciousness has two components: wakefulness and awareness (2). Awareness is "the ability to have, and the having of, experience of any kind" (2). We humans are "typically aware of our surroundings and of bodily sensations, but the contents of awareness can also include our memories, thoughts, emotions and intentions" (2).

Perhaps the most commonly known disorder of consciousness is *coma*. In a coma, a patient's eyes remain closed, and the person appears to be asleep but cannot be aroused (3, 4). A patient in a coma lacks both wakefulness and awareness (5). A patient in a *vegetative state* (VS), on the other hand, is awake but unaware. Vegetative state patients exhibit sleep-wake cycles but show no awareness of self or their environment when awake (6). A vegetative state has been distinguished from a *minimally conscious state* (MCS), in which a patient "demonstrates unequivocal but fluctuating evidence of awareness of self and the environment" (5). Some vegetative state patients move into a minimally conscious state (5). Neither condition should be confused with *locked-in syndrome*, "a rare neurological disorder characterized by complete paralysis of voluntary muscles in all parts of the body except for those that control eye movements" (7). Individuals suffering from this disorder "are conscious and can think and reason, but are unable to speak or move" (7).

In the recent literature on the vegetative state, question has been raised about the appropriateness of the term itself. The term "vegetative state" was originally chosen to name the condition in question because "*to vegetate* is defined in the Oxford English dictionary as 'to live a merely physical life, devoid of intellectual activity or social intercourse (1740)' and *vegetative* is used to describe 'an organic body capable of growth and development but devoid of sensation and thought (1764)'" (8). However, some have taken this terminology in a pejorative sense, prompting affirmations that a human being, "*even if seriously ill or disabled in the exercise of his highest functions, is and always will be a man*, and he will never become a 'vegetable' or an 'animal'" (9). Concomitantly, it is affirmed that "the intrinsic value and personal dignity of every human being do not change, no matter what the concrete circumstances of his or her life" (9). Thus the terminology *unresponsive wakefulness syndrome* (UWS) has been suggested for the condition in question (10, 11). Our continued use of the term "vegetative state" reflects terminology embedded in a vast amount of medical literature and is not intended to carry a negative connotation about the human status and dignity of patients in this condition.

Ethically, there has been a particular focus on the appropriate medical treatment of patients in a vegetative state. We will begin with a description of conventional medical views about the vegetative state, and then explore recent medical research on this condition. This factual information will lead into consideration of the ethical issues surrounding treatment of patients in a vegetative state.

The Vegetative State: Conventional Views

In the 1990s, a Multi-Society Task Force on PVS, sponsored by five different American medical societies, proposed the following criteria for diagnosing a vegetative state:

- The patient gives no evidence of being aware of self or the environment, and is unable to interact with others.
- The patient gives no evidence of sustained, reproducible, purposeful, or voluntary behavioral responses to stimuli.
- The patient gives no evidence of understanding or using language.
- The patient goes through sleep-wake cycles.
- The brain functions of the hypothalamus and brain stem are sufficiently preserved to allow the patient to survive with medical and nursing care.
- The patient has incontinence of both bowel and bladder.
- Cranial-nerve reflexes (e.g., reaction of the pupils to light, the gag reflex) and spinal reflexes are preserved in varying degrees (3, 4).

A patient in a vegetative state may occasionally grunt, scream, smile, or shed tears, and show movement of nonparalyzed limbs (3, 4). While most vegetative state patients show some response to painful stimuli (e.g., limb withdrawal, facial grimacing, groaning, rise in respiratory and pulse rates, and blood pressure), it has been thought that "these responses are all at reflex level and do not indicate that pain is being experienced at a conscious level" (8). Most patients in a vegetative state who survive for a long time are able to breathe on their own and have a functioning cardiovascular system (3).

A *persistent vegetative state* (PVS) is defined as a vegetative state which has continued for at least 1 month. It can occur after an acute traumatic brain injury (e.g., an injury due to a car accident) or after an acute nontraumatic brain injury (e.g., cardiac arrest). It can be caused by degenerative or metabolic disorders (e.g., Alzheimer's disease, Parkinson's disease, Huntington's disease) or by developmental malformations in infants and children (e.g., anencephalic infants in whom part of the brain never develops) (3, 4). Sometimes a patient in a persistent vegetative state because of an acute traumatic or nontraumatic brain injury will regain consciousness and abilities to function in various ways (12).

A patient in a persistent vegetative state is said to enter a *permanent vegetative state* when the diagnosis is that the condition is irreversible and the chance that the patient will regain consciousness is very, very small (3, 4). In the case of a traumatic brain injury, a persistent vegetative state is considered permanent 12 months after the injury in both adults and children. If the persistent vegetative state is related to a nontraumatic injury, it is considered permanent after 3 months in both adults and children (12). Patients who are in a vegetative state due to degenerative or metabolic diseases have no possibility of recovery (12). For infants and children with brain malformations severe enough to cause developmental vegetative states, lack of consciousness by the age of 6 months almost completely precludes the potential for future improvement (12). In the case of anencephalic infants, it is clear at birth that there is no possibility for recovery because the complete absence of the cerebral cortex of the brain precludes consciousness (12).

In the case of brain injury, the Multi-Society Task Force on PVS reported the average life expectancy of such patients as 2–5 years (12). However, a very small number of patients "have survived for more than 15 years . . . including three patients who survived for more than 17, 37, and 41 years" (12). Reported causes of death for patients in a persistent or permanent vegetative state have included pulmonary or urinary tract infection, generalized systemic failure, respiratory failure, and recurrent strokes or tumors (12).

The Vegetative State: Recent Research

Standard diagnostic criteria for the vegetative state have been based on observation of the patient's behavior (13). Commenting on this fact, the 2003 report of the Royal College of Physicians on the vegetative state states that "as our techniques of assessment are fallible, we can never exclude the possibility of some awareness with complete certainty" which "leaves open the possibility that some extremely simple forms of awareness may survive in the VS" (2).

Going beyond the observable behavior of vegetative state patients, neuroimaging is now being used in studying these patients, with the following results:

> Both functional magnetic resonance imaging (fMRI) and electroencephalography (EEG) have been used to detect residual cognitive function and even conscious awareness in vegetative and minimally conscious patients. . . . Indeed, neuroimaging has shown that a subset of this patient group (17–19%), who consistently satisfy the behavioral diagnostic criteria of the vegetative state, retain conscious awareness undetectable through beside clinical examination. (6)

One type of testing of patients involves mental imagery tasks. In one study using this technique, a patient who fulfilled all of the clinical criteria for the vegetative state was placed in an MRI scanner and "asked to imagine hitting a tennis ball back and forth to an imaginary coach when she heard the word 'tennis' and to imagine walking from room to room in her house when she heard the word 'house'" (14). A group of healthy control volunteers underwent the same procedure, with distinct areas of the brain consistently being activated for each imagery task (14). Significantly, "the fMRI responses in the patient were indistinguishable from those observed in the control volunteers in both tasks" (14). This indicated that the patient had retained the ability to understand and respond to spoken commands, and concomitantly, that she was consciously aware (14). A subsequent study using the same mental imagery tasks "demonstrated that, out of a group of 23 patients in a vegetative state, 4 were able to generate similarly reliable fMRI responses to commands and were therefore also covertly aware" (14; see also 15).

Further, the mental imagery task was modified to achieve communication with vegetative state patients (16). Patient and control subjects were asked a "yes" or "no" question and instructed to respond by using one type of mental imagery for "yes" and the other for "no" (14–16). One notable case involves a patient who had been repeatedly diagnosed as in a vegetative state for 12 years after a traumatic brain injury, well beyond the point at which the vegetative state would be considered permanent (14). This patient "was able to provide correct answers to multiple externally verifiable questions, including his own name, the name of his personal support worker (who he had only encountered in the years following his accident) and the current date" (14).

Yet other tests have indicated awareness and cognitive functioning in some vegetative state patients. Both functional MRI and EEG have been used in this testing (17, 18) which has involved such tasks as selective attention to auditory stimuli (19), counting how many times a particular word ("yes" or "no") occurs in a series of words (20), and face recognition and emotion (21). We will subsequently consider the ethical implications of these recent research findings.

Various therapies are under trial to promote recovery of function, to whatever level possible, in patients in a vegetative state due to brain injuries (22). These therapies include deep brain stimulation (23), electrical stimulation of the dorsal column (24), pharmacological agents (25–29), and stem cell therapy (30). Attempts are also being made to identify prognostic markers for recovery (31–33).

Life-Sustaining Treatments for Vegetative State Patients

A patient in a persistent or permanent vegetative state needs various kinds of care:

> Preventive care is foremost. Daily exercises in a range of movements slow the formation of limb contractures, which otherwise become particularly severe in patients in a persistent vegetative state. Daily skin care and frequent repositioning of the patient prevent decubitus ulcers. A tracheostomy may be required to maintain airway patency and prevent aspiration pneumonia. Bladder and bowel care is desirable for hygienic reasons. Since pulmonary and urinary tract infections are common, appropriate monitoring and, if necessary, treatment with antibiotics are required. Placement of nasogastric, gastrostomy, or jejunostomy feeding tubes is usually necessary to maintain adequate nutrition and hydration. (12)

Potentially, other procedures or treatments might be added if they become necessary for prolonging life: diagnostic tests, blood or blood product transfusions, transfer to the intensive care unit (ICU, dialysis, chemotherapy for cancer, minor surgery, major surgery, mechanical ventilation, cardiopulmonary resuscitation, organ transplantation (12, 34).

The focus of our discussion will be on the ethics of using or forgoing life-sustaining treatments for patients in a persistent or permanent vegetative state, and on the particular ethical questions which have arisen for this category of patients.

As evidenced by the highly publicized court cases involving Nancy Cruzan and Terri Schiavo (1), the withdrawal of assisted nutrition and hydration from patients in a vegetative state has been particularly controversial. According to the principle of weighing benefits and burdens (see Chapter 6, "Making Decisions about Using or Forgoing Life-Sustaining Treatments"), such withdrawal is clearly permissible if assisted nutrition and hydration proves useless or futile, providing no benefit to the patient, or if it proves more burdensome than beneficial. Thus, the principle of weighing benefits and burdens would justify withdrawing assisted nutrition and hydration from a patient in a persistent or permanent vegetative state if the feeding tube does not work because the tube itself has developed complications such as infection or bleeding, or because it has become tangled in the bowels so that the bowel tissue dies and can no longer absorb nutrients (35). Or again, this ethical principle could justify withdrawing assisted nutrition and hydration on grounds of excessive burdens if the vegetative state patient experiences recurrent pneumonia caused by feedings going up the food pipe and down the windpipe (35). The same would hold true if the feeding tube is involved in complications such as causing diarrhea that has resulted in infected ulcers, or causing electrolyte abnormalities that has led to seizures (35).

Some have seen the diagnosis of permanency of a vegetative state as ethically significant in terms of the obligation to provide assisted nutrition and hydration. Specifically, some have maintained that "once a firm prognosis of permanent unconsciousness has been made, A[ssisted] H[ydration] N[utrition] may be removed" because it offers no hope of benefit to the patient (36). This position is based on the beliefs that the purpose of health care is "to enable people to strive for the purpose of life, not merely to function at the biological level" and that pursuing the purpose of life "requires cognitive-affective function" (36). On the other hand, based on the view that providing nutrition and hydration to patients (even by artificial means) is part of the normal care due to the sick person and not a special medical treatment (9), others have maintained that the permanency of the vegetative state does not in itself justify withdrawal of assisted nutrition and hydration (9, 37). Nevertheless, those who espouse this position would allow withdrawal of assisted nutrition and hydration from a patient in a permanent vegetative state if the procedure cannot reasonably be expected to prolong the patient's life or if it proves excessively burdensome for the patient (37).

When artificial nutrition and hydration are withdrawn, patients in a persistent or permanent vegetative state usually die within 10–14 days. Dehydration and electrolyte imbalance, rather than malnutrition, are the immediate causes of death. Except for dryness of the skin and mucous membranes, it is not readily apparent to family members that the patient is dying of dehydration. Further, appropriate nursing care can prevent these signs of dehydration. Facial swelling can occur as a result of prolonged administration of artificial nutrition and hydration but, as the patient becomes dehydrated, this swelling decreases and facial features may assume a more normal appearance during the last few days of life (12). The Royal College of Physicians has recommended that, in virtue of the element of uncertainty as to whether a vegetative state patient is wholly unaware, "it is reasonable to administer sedation when hydration and nutrition are withdrawn to eliminate the possibility of suffering, however remote" (2). Further, it is recommended that "the normal standards of palliative care should be observed to ensure the dignity of the death" (2).

One challenge in making decisions about using or forgoing life-sustaining treatments (such as the use of antibiotics in the case of infection) for patients in a vegetative state is the phenomenon of late recovery from the vegetative state, even after the time period for diagnosis of permanency of the condition has passed. Although such recovered patients may be left with severe disability (38, 39), this is not universally true. Late recovery with only moderate disability is possible (39). For example, a case has been recorded of a 22-year-old male student who recovered consciousness from a vegetative state 19 months after a traumatic brain injury. A further slow recovery of motor and cognitive functions was observed in him over a period of 7 years after the brain injury. The patient progressed to the point of being able to live in the community, speaking, walking, and undertaking daily living as well as outdoor leisure activities independently. In fact, he was able to resume his previous university studies and undertake a part-time noncompetitive job (39).

Another significant challenge in making decisions about using or forgoing life-sustaining treatments for patients in a vegetative state is the discovery of awareness and cognitive function in some of these patients, even in patients considered to be in a permanent vegetative state (see above). This concern is exacerbated by uncertainty regarding the extent to which vegetative state patients as a class retain awareness and cognitive functioning. In the case of neuroimaging studies, successful completion of the assigned tasks by a patient "allows researchers to be highly confident that the participant possesses awareness" (16). On the other hand, a negative test result—the failure to detect awareness and cognitive function—is ambiguous. It could mean that the patient in fact lacks awareness (14, 16) or it could be the result of a failure in the test conditions (16). Specifically, the patient may fail to hear or understand the instructions, have low levels of arousal, fall asleep during the test, or move frequently thereby preventing researchers from obtaining brain images suitable for analysis (14, 16). Or again, "the neuroimaging methods used may simply be insensitive to small changes in brain activity in some patients" (14). In sum, "no conclusions or claims about the preservation or loss of residual awareness in patients can be drawn on the basis of a negative finding" (14).

In any case, the discovery of awareness and cognitive function in some vegetative state patients has raised the issue of the ethical significance of consciousness in making decisions about using or forgoing life-sustaining treatments (6, 14, 40). On the one hand, "evidence of consciousness . . . is thought by some to be a reason not to withdraw LSTs [life-sustaining treatments]" (6). On the other hand, it has been argued that "'enjoyment of consciousness might actually give stronger moral reasons not to preserve a patient's life'" should the patient be experiencing great physical or mental suffering (14). The question is a complex one which will require further study and discussion:

> consciousness does not preclude withdrawal of life-sustaining treatment. It is ethical to withdraw life-sustaining treatment even from patients who are fully conscious, for example when the patient requests it, when the treatment is futile, or when the burdens of treatment outweigh their benefits. Neuroimaging might indicate that a patient who appears to be in a vegetative state is actually fully conscious and "locked-in." Whereas it might be thought that we are morally required to do our best to preserve the life of a patient in this state, some might ask whether such a life is worse than death. A number of patients with LIS [Locked-in Syndrome] express a desire not to go on living and some request euthanasia. On the other hand the capacity of humans to adapt to their condition, no matter how adverse, has been amply documented in other contexts. Indeed, the self-scored perception of mental wellbeing in one survey of patients in LIS was not significantly lower than that of age-matched normal subjects. However, surveys of patients able to communicate may not be relevant to a more severely affected population of patients with full LIS and an apparent vegetative state. Many may also have been in such a state for a long time. Their situation might be compared unfavourably with the worst form of solitary confinement in prison. It is not necessarily clear, on the basis of the best interests of such patients, that life-sustaining treatment should be continued. This is a subject that requires further active debate. (40)

Given that fMRI has succeeded in establishing some communication with vegetative state patients (see above), there has been speculation about the possibility of using fMRI to "give such patients the chance to voice their own opinion about the continuation or withdrawal of life-sustaining treatment" (40). Ethically, this plan would be supported by the principle of autonomy. However, in considering this theoretical possibility, question has been raised about establishing the decision making capacity of such patients (6) and at the level required to "make complex decisions about their care" (41).

Case Study Revisited

How does our discussion apply to the hypothetical case of Carla Munoz presented at the beginning of the chapter?

Carla is presently incapacitated to make health care decisions. Thus, it falls to a proxy decision maker to make those decisions on her behalf. There is no indication in the case study that she has legally appointed someone as her proxy decision maker through a durable power of attorney for health care. Her husband Lucas would normally serve as her proxy decision maker.

Immediately at issue is whether antibiotics should be administered for Carla's pneumonia. Lucas' immediate reaction is to "insist that antibiotics—and any other treatment medically indicated—be provided for his wife." Carla is also receiving medically assisted nutrition and hydration.

As the proxy decision maker, Lucas should employ the principle of substituted judgment as an extension of patient autonomy, attempting to reach the decision that Carla would make if she were able to make a decision (see Chapter 8). Since the principle of weighing benefits and burdens ought to guide an individual's decision making about medical treatments (see Chapter 7), Lucas should ask the questions: How would Carla view the benefits and burdens of antibiotics to cure her pneumonia, and how would she view the benefits and burdens of assisted nutrition and hydration?

Carla has been in a vegetative state for seven weeks, which places her in the category of being in a "persistent" vegetative state. Her vegetative state is the result of a traumatic brain injury (a car accident). According to the report of the Royal College of Physicians, "people in a VS [vegetative state] one month after trauma stand a slightly better than even chance of regaining awareness" (2). Furthermore, various therapies are under trial to promote recovery of function in patients in a vegetative state due to brain injuries, and these might be tried with Carla. These considerations argue in favor of administering the antibiotics (and other medically indicated life-sustaining treatments) to Carla—as her husband wishes—to allow the possibility of recovery. Life-sustaining treatments are a benefit to Carla in this respect, a benefit we can presume she would want. Moreover, the tube feeding is apparently working and there is no indication that the procedure is causing problems for her (burdens) which would justify withdrawing the medically assisted nutrition and hydration.

Now let us suppose that the worst case scenario occurs and that, 12 months after the car accident, Carla still remains in a vegetative state. According to conventional views of the vegetative state, her condition can now be diagnosed as "permanent." And let us further suppose that she again develops pneumonia. Should antibiotics be administered? This decision is more complex to make.

One complicating factor is the phenomenon of late recovery from a vegetative state, including a permanent vegetative state, with severe to only moderate disability. Using the principle of substituted judgment, Lucas will have to determine if Carla is the kind of person who would want to be kept alive to take this chance.

Another complicating factor is the possibility of covert awareness and cognitive function in Carla. Lucas would need to think about how Carla would feel about living in this kind of condition. In explicating the principle of weighing benefits and burdens, we noted that some ethicists advocate looking at "the well-being of the whole person" and not merely at the benefits of treatment to a particular organ when making decisions about using or forgoing life-sustaining treatments. On this view, a particular medical treatment may ameliorate a particular physical malady but, given the patient's overall medical condition, may not really be a benefit to the patient (see Chapter 7).

CHAPTER SUMMARY

Key Terms and Concepts

vegetative state: a disorder of consciousness in which the patient is awake but unaware.

persistent vegetative state: a vegetative state that has continued for at least one month.

permanent vegetative state: a vegetative state that is diagnosed as irreversible and where the chance that the patient will regain unconsciousness is very, very small.

principle of patient autonomy: self-determination; an individual's right to hold views, make choices, and take actions based on personal values and beliefs.

principle of substituted judgment: a proxy decision maker attempts to reach the decision that the incapacitated patient would make if he or she were able to choose, relying on written or oral directives explicitly given by the patient or on knowledge of the patient's beliefs, values, preferences, and life-long behavior patterns.

principle of weighing benefits and burdens: A life-sustaining treatment ought to be used if it provides more benefits than burdens. It is morally permissible to forgo (that is, withhold or withdraw) a life-sustaining treatment if the burdens of the treatment outweigh its benefits or if the treatment is useless or futile.

Key Points

- Conventional medical views of the vegetative state are being modified by research which indicates that at least some vegetative state patients retain some degree of awareness and cognitive function. Various therapies are also under trial to promote recovery of function of vegetative state patients.
- A patient in a persistent or permanent vegetative state needs routine nursing care (e.g., skin care, repositioning, bladder, and bowel care). In addition, treatment decisions will have to be made about using or forgoing assisted nutrition and hydration (tube feeding), and perhaps about such treatments and procedures as antibiotics, diagnostic tests, blood or blood product transfusions, transfer to the ICU, dialysis, chemotherapy, surgery, ventilators, and resuscitation.
- Controversy has surrounded the withdrawal of assisted nutrition and hydration from a vegetative state patient, especially those diagnosed as being in a permanent vegetative state.
- Decisions about using or forgoing life-sustaining treatments for patients in a vegetative state, including those diagnosed as being in a permanent vegetative state, are complicated by the phenomenon of late recovery from the vegetative state and the discovery of awareness and cognitive function in some of these patients.
- In making medical treatment decisions for patients in a vegetative state, the proxy decision maker should be guided by the principle of substituted judgment (an extension of patient autonomy) and by the principle of weighing benefits and burdens.

FOR FURTHER DISCUSSION

Suppose that you are the allied health representative on your facility's ethics committee, and that the following cases involving vegetative state patients are brought to the committee for an ethics consult. The following options are available:

1. Continue routine nursing care, but stop all treatments necessary for prolonging life, including assisted nutrition and hydration.
2. Continue assisted nutrition and hydration as well as routine nursing care, but do not add any additional procedures or treatments.
3. Continue assisted nutrition and hydration as well as routine nursing care, and in addition add (some or all of) such treatments as the following if they become necessary for prolonging life: antibiotics, simple diagnostic tests, blood or blood product transfusions, transfer to the intensive care unit, dialysis, chemotherapy for cancer, minor surgery, major surgery, mechanical ventilation, cardiopulmonary resuscitation, organ transplantation.
4. Other (describe) (12, 34).

Case 1. Patricia Farrell, 33, has been diagnosed as being in a permanent vegetative state. Since she became unconscious after a car accident 15 months ago, Patricia has been on assisted nutrition and hydration. Recently she has developed aspiration pneumonia from the feeding tube. Patricia's physician, Dr. Eileen Swanson, speaks with her husband Richard, and recommends against the use of antibiotics. Indeed Dr. Swanson mentions to Richard that perhaps it is time to think about removing the feeding tube as well. Richard, however, insists that the doctor "do everything" to save his wife. Richard admits that, after the death of her father, Patricia had stated quite clearly that she herself wanted to "go quickly" and did not wish to linger on for several years in a debilitated state, as had happened to her father. Nevertheless, Richard says that "miracles can happen," and that he just doesn't feel right about "giving up" on Patricia at this point. Because Dr. Swanson is concerned that Richard has false hopes for his wife, she encourages him to meet with the facility's ethics committee to talk about the situation.

Case 2. Consider again the case of Patricia Farrell, with the following change of circumstances: Richard relates that, after the death of her father, Patricia had stated quite clearly that, if anything happened to her so that she could not take care of herself, she did not want anything done to shorten or prematurely take her life, as she believed had happened to her father while in the hospital.

Case 3. Two months ago Tom McGann, 45, suffered a serious a brain injury in a car accident. Since that time he has been unconscious, and a neurologist has told his wife, Alice, that he is in a persistent vegetative state. Assisted nutrition and hydration has been used during this time to sustain his life. Tom has recently developed kidney problems, and Alice must now make a decision about dialysis. Tom had always been very active physically, golfing, bowling, and taking long bicycle rides on nature trails. Because of this, Alice feels that Tom would never want to continue to exist in an unconscious state, confined to bed, and not able to do any of the things he enjoyed about life. Kidney failure, Alice believes, may be a blessing in disguise, "letting her husband go free." Alice tells her husband's doctor that dialysis should not be started. However, because this decision will ensure that Tom will die, the doctor encourages Alice to talk with the facility's ethics committee before she makes the final decision.

For each case:

- *Go through the case on your own. Write down the medical facts and ethical principles you think should enter into the conversation with the proxy decision maker.*
- *Share your thoughts about the case with other members of the class (as you would with other members of the ethics committee on which you serve and with the proxy decision maker). This may be done either in small groups or with the class as a whole.*
- *Now imagine yourself as the proxy decision maker. After having had a conversation with the members of the ethics committee, what course of action would you decide to take, and why? Is there agreement or disagreement among the members of the class?*

References

1. Gregory E. Pence, *Classic Cases in Medical Ethics*, 5th ed. (New York: McGraw–Hill, 2007).
2. Royal College of Physicians, "The Vegetative State: Guidance on Diagnosis and Management," *Clinical Medicine* 3/3 (May/June 2003): 249–54.
3. The Multi-Society Task Force on PVS, "Medical Aspects of the Persistent Vegetative State," Part One, *New England Journal of Medicine* 330/21 (May 26, 1994):1499–1508.
4. American Neurological Association Committee on Ethical Affairs, "Persistent Vegetative State: Report of the American Neurological Association Committee on Ethical Affairs," *Annals of Neurology* 33/4 (April 1993): 386–90.

5. Norman Ford, "Understanding the Persistent Vegetative State and the Ethics of Care for Its Patients," *The Australian Catholic Record* 92/3 (July 2015): 317–29.

6. Charles Weijer, Andrew Peterson, Fiona Webster, Mackenzie Graham, Damian Cruse, Davinia Fernandez-Espejo, Teneille Gofton, Laura E. Gonzalez-Lara, Andrea Lazosky, Lorina Naci, Loretta Norton, Kathy Speechley, Bryan Young and Adrian M. Owen, "Ethics of Neuroimaging After Serious Brain Injury," *BMC Medical Ethics* 15/41 (May 20, 2014): 1–13.

7. National Institute of Neurological Disorders and Stroke, National Institutes of Health, "*Locked-in Syndrome Information Page.*" http://www.ninds.nih.gov/disorders/lockedinsyndrome/lockedinsyndrome.htm. Accessed January 2016.

8. Bryan Jennett, *The Vegetative State Medical Facts, Ethical And Legal Dilemmas* (New York: Cambridge University Press, 2002).

9. Pope John Paul II, "To the Participants in the International Congress on 'Life-Sustaining Treatments and Vegetative State: Scientific Advances and Ethical Dilemmas,'" in *The Case of Terri Schiavo Ethics at the End of Life*, eds. Arthur L. Caplan, James J. McCartney, and Dominic Sisti (Amherst, NY: Prometheus Books, 2006).

10. S. Laureys, G.G. Celesia, F. Cohadon, J. Lavrijsen, J. Leon-Carrion, W.G. Sannita, L. Sazbon, E. Schmutzhard, K.R. von Wild, A. Zeman, G. Dolce; European Task Force on Disorders of Consciousness, "Unresponsive Wakefulness Syndrome: A New Name for the Vegetative or Apallic Syndrome," *BioMed Central Medicine* 8/68 (2010).

11. K. von Wild, S.T. Laureys, F. Gerstenbrand, G. Dolce, and G. Onose, "The Vegetative State—A Syndrome in Search of a Name," *Journal of Medicine and Life* 5/1 (January–March 2012): 3–15.

12. Multi-Society Task Force on PVS, "Medical Aspects of the Persistent Vegetative State," Part Two, *New England Journal of Medicine* 330/22 (June 2, 1994): 1572–79.

13. Katja Kuehlmeyer, Nicole Palmour, Richard J. Riopelle, James L. Bernat, Ralf J. Jox and Eric Racine, "Physicians' Attitudes Toward Medical and Ethical Challenges for Patients in the Vegetative State: Comparing Canadian and German Perspectives in a Vignette Survey," *BMC Neurology* 14/1 (2014): 1–18.

14. Davinia Fernandez-Espejo and Andrian M. Owen, "Detecting Awareness After Severe Brain Injury," *Nature Reviews Neuroscience* 14 (November 2013): 1–9.

15. Martin M. Monti, Audrey Vanhaudenhuyse, Martin M. Coleman, Melanie Boly, John D. Pickard, Luaba Tshibanda, Adrian M. Owen, and

Steven Laureys, "Willful Modulation of Brain Activity in Disorders of Consciousness," *New England Journal of Medicine* 362/7 (February 18, 2010): 579–89.

16. Mackenzie Graham, Charles Weijer, Andrew Peterson, Lorina Naci, Damian Cruse, Davinia Fernandez-Espejo, Laura Gonzalez-Lara, and Adrian M. Owen, "Acknowledging Awareness: Informing Families of Individual Research Results for Patients in the Vegetative State," *Journal of Medical Ethics Online First* (July 30, 2014): 1–5.

17. Laura Bell, "Locked Inside," *Science News* 188/3 (August 8, 2015): 18–21.

18. Srivas Chennu, Paola Finoia, Evelyn Kamau, Judith Allanson, Guy B. Williams, Martin M. Monti, Valdas Noreika, Aurina Arnatkeviciute, Andres Canales-Johnson, Francisco Olivares, Daniela Cabezas-Soto, David K. Menon, John D. Pickard, Adrian M. Owen, and Tristan A. Bekinschtein, "Spectral Signatures of Reorganised Brain Networks in Disorders of Consciousness," *PLoS Computational Biology* 10/10 (October 2014): 1–16.

19. Lorina Naci and Adrian M. Own, "Making Every Word Count for Nonresponsive Patients," *JAMA Neurology* 70/10 (2013): 1235–41.

20. Srivas Chennu, Paola Finola, Evelyn Kamau, Martin M. Monti, Judith Allanson, John D. Pickard, Adrian M. Owen, Tristan A. Bekinschtein, 'Dissociable Endogenous and Exogenous Attention in Disorders of Consciousness," *Neuroimage: Clinical* 3 (2013): 450–61.

21. Haggai Sharon, Yotam Pasternak, Eti Ben Simon, Michal Gruberger, Nir Giladi, Ben Zion Krimchanski, David Hassin, and Talma Hendler, "Emotional Processing of Personally Familiar Faces in the Vegetative State," *PLoS One* 8/9 (September 2013): 1–8.

22. Mohammad Yousuf Rathor, Mohammad Fauzi Abdul Rani, Tarmizi Che Abdullah Shahrin, and Hasnur Zaman Hashim, "Persistent Vegetative State After Traumatic Brain Injury A Case Report and Review of the Literature," *Bangladesh Journal of Medical Science* 13/3 (July 2014): 358–65.

23. Sara Patuzzo and Paolo Manganotti, "Deep Brain Stimulation in Persistent Vegetative States: Ethical Issues Governing Decision Making," *Behavioural Neurology* 2014 (2014): 1—6.

24. T. Yokoyama, Y. Kamei, M. Shoda, M. Abe, K. Onouchi, A. Kasama, T. Inoue and T. Kanno, "Treatment of Vegetative Status With Dorsal Column Stimulation," *No Shinkei Geka* 18/1 (January 1990): 39–45.

25. Francesca Pistois, R. Mura, S. Govoni, M. Fini, and M. Sara, "Awakenings and Awareness Recovery in Disorders of Consciousness: Is There a Role for Drugs?" *CNS Drugs* 24/8 (Aug. 2010): 625–38.

26. R. Ciurleo, P. Bramanti, and R.S. Calabro, "Pharmacotherapy for Disorders of Consciousness: re 'Awakening' Drugs Really a Possibility?" *Drugs* 73/17 (November 2013): 1849–62.

27. BZ Krimchansky, O. Keren, L. Sazbon and Z. Groswasser, "Differential Time and Related Appearance of Signs, Indicating Improvement in the State of Consciousness in Vegetative State Traumatic Brain Injury (Vs-Tbi) Patients After Initiation of Dopamine Treatment," *Brain Injury* 18/11 (November 2004): 1099–105.

28. Wakoto Matsuda, Yoji Komatsu, Kiyoyuki Yanaka, and Akira Matsumura, "Levodopa Treatment for Patients in Persistent Vegetative or Minimally Conscious States," *Neuropsychological Rehabilitation* 15/3-4 (2005): 41427.

29. W. Matsuda, A. Matsumura, Y. Komatsu, K. Yanaka and T. Nose, "Awakenings From Persistent Vegetative State: Report of Three Cases With Parkinsonism and Brain Stem Lesions on MRI," *Journal of Neurology, Neurosurgery & Psychiatry* 74 (2003): 1571–3.

30. Chunlei Tian, Xiongwei Wang, Xiaodan Wang, Lei Wang, Xuguang Wang, Shengmei Wu, and Zhixian Wan, "Autologous Bone Marrow Mesenchymal Stem Cell Therapy in the Subacute Stage of Traumatic Brain Injury by Lumbar Puncture," *Experimental and Clinical Transplantation* 11/2 (April 2013): 176–81.

31. A. Estraneo, P. Moretta, V. Loreto, B. Lanzillo, A. Cozzolino, A. Saltalamacchia, F. Lullo, L. Santoro, and L. Trojano, "Predictors of Recovery of Responsiveness in Prolonged Anoxic Vegetative State," *Neurology* 80/5 (January 29, 2013): 464–70.

32. Xiao G. Kang, Li Li, Dong Wei, Xiao-Xia Xu, Rui Zhao, Yun-Yun Jing, Ying-Ying Su, Li-Ze Xiong, Gang Zhao, and Wen Jiang, "Development of a Simple Score to Predict Outcome for Unresponsive Wakefulness Syndrome," *Critical Care* 18/1 (February 26, 2014): R37.

33. Dominik Vogel, Alexandra Markl, Tao Yu, Boris Kotchoubey, Simone Lang, and Friedemann Muller, "Can Mental Imagery Functional Magnetic Resonance Imaging Predict Recovery in Patients With Disorders of Consciousness?" *Archives of Physical Medicine and Rehabilitation* 94/10 (October 2013): 1891–98.

34. Ellen Fox and Carol Stocking, "Ethics Consultants' Recommendations for Life-Prolonging Treatment of Patients in a Persistent Vegetative State," *Journal of the American Medical Association* 270/21 (December 1, 1993): 2578–82.

35. Daniel P. Sulmasy, "Preserving Life? The Vatican & PVS," *Commonweal* 134/21 (December 7, 2007): 16–18.

36. Kevin O'Rourke and Patrick Norris, "Care of PVS Patients Catholic Opinion in the United States" in *The Case of Terri Schiavo Ethics at the End of Life*, eds. Arthur L. Caplan, James J. McCartney, and Dominic A. Sisti (Amherst, NY: Prometheus Books, 2006).

37. United States Conference of Catholic Bishops, *Ethical and Religious Directives for Catholic Health Care Services*, 5th ed., No. 58. http://www.usccb.org. Accessed January 2016.

38. A. Estraneo, P. Moretta, V. Loreto, B. Lanzillo, L. Santoro and L. Trojano, "Late Recovery After Traumatic, Anoxic, or Hemorrhagic Long-Lasting Vegetative State," *Neurology* 75/3 (July 20, 2010): 239–45.

39. E. Sancisi, A. Battistini, C. Di Stefano, L. Simoncini, L. Simoncini, P. Montagna, and R. Piperno, "Late Recovery From Post-Traumatic Vegetative State," *Brain Injury* 23/2 (February 2009): 163–66.

40. D.J. Wilkinson, G. Kahane, M. Horne, and J. Savulescu, "Functional Neuroimaging and Withdrawal of Life-Sustaining Treatment From Vegetative Patients," *Journal of Medical Ethics* 35 (2009): 508–11.

41. Katie Drummond, "Gray Area: Unraveling the Inner Worlds of Vegetative State Patients," *The Verge* (November 7, 2013). http://www.theverge.com/2013/11/7/5074718/vegetative-state-patients-awareness-neuroimaging. Accessed January 2016.

Chapter 11

Euthanasia and Physician Aid-in-Dying

Euthanasia and physician aid-in-dying (also known as physician-assisted suicide) are both deliberate attempts to end a patient's life in order to end his or her suffering. These practices differ in the agent who introduces the immediate and direct cause of death. The act is called *euthanasia* when a person other than the patient directly does something to cause the patient's death. If a doctor injects a patient with a lethal drug with the intent of bringing about the patient's death (perhaps in response to the patient's request), this is an act of euthanasia. *Physician aid-in-dying* takes place when a physician provides the patient with the means to take his or her own life but the patient is the one who directly initiates the action causing death. Typically, a doctor deliberately prescribes medication that a patient can take at home to cause his death. (For the distinction between these practices and forgoing life-sustaining treatments, see Chapter 7.)

Euthanasia is considered *voluntary* when it is undertaken at the request of or with the consent of the patient; *involuntary*, then it is performed without the patient's consent. If a patient who is physically unable to take his own life asks a doctor to administer a lethal drug which will cause his death, this is an instance of voluntary euthanasia. If a physician administers a death producing drug to an elderly dementia patient solely at the request of the patient's children, this is a case of involuntary euthanasia.

Physician aid-in-dying or euthanasia might be considered when the patient is in the final stages of the dying process, or when the patient has a progressively debilitating disease, or when the patient has a terminal condition or a severely debilitating disease and is experiencing intense suffering.

Euthanasia as well as physician aid-in-dying is allowed in Belgium, the Netherlands, and Luxembourg (1). As of early 2016, euthanasia is not legally allowed in any state in the United States but physician aid-in-dying is allowed in the states of Oregon, Washington, Montana, Vermont, and California (2).

In this chapter you will learn about:

- The provisions of laws allowing physician aid-in-dying;
- Arguments presented in favor of euthanasia and physician aid-in-dying;
- Objections raised against euthanasia and physician aid-in-dying;
- Pain management and palliative sedation.

Case Study

Mark Bennett has just finished his training as a physician assistant. Shortly after beginning work at Parkview Memorial Hospital, he encounters a situation he finds very disturbing.

Ruth and Tom Jackson have been married for over 40 years. Three years ago, Ruth was found to have stomach and colon cancer. Since that time, she has undergone chemotherapy treatment. However, it was recently discovered that the cancer has spread to Ruth's pancreas.

Ruth has now been hospitalized at Parkview for a week. Her weight is down to 95 pounds, and friends who come to see her remark how much she has "aged." Her pain is constant. Although Ruth is receiving pain medication, it doesn't seem strong enough to really help her.

Tom spent last night at the hospital at his wife's side. Her discomfort was so intense that she kept waking up and wasn't able to sleep well. All Tom could do was sit and hold her hand while she twisted and turned in bed. Several times during the night, Ruth moaned that she wished "it was over."

The next morning Tom asks to talk with PA Mark Bennett. The Jackson and Bennett families have been friends for years, and Tom knew Mark as he was growing up. Tom feels Mark will understand what Ruth is going through.

"I know you can give injections of medications," Tom tells Mark. "I want you to get several doses of Ruth's pain medication, and give it to her all at once to end her suffering. If you don't do this, I will take a pillow and smother Ruth. She's going to die anyway, and I love her too much to allow her to suffer any more."

If something is not done, Mark fears that Tom will carry out his threat to smother his wife, with dire legal consequences for him. Mark begins to think about what the options are in this case.

* * *

At age 65, Christopher Vaughn decides to sell the jewelry store he started and managed for 40 years in a small Midwestern community. The first 2 years of his retirement are good ones, giving him the opportunity to spend time with his six grandchildren. But then his wife, Roberta, begins to notice behavioral changes in him. After he "got lost" driving home one afternoon, they both agree that he should be checked out medically. It is learned that Christopher is in the very early stages of Alzheimer's disease.

To make matters worse, Roberta dies unexpectedly. Christopher decides to enter Glenview Village, a multilevel facility, in order to "prepare for the future." Initially, Christopher resides in an assisted living apartment, but he understands what is to come as the disease progresses. And, apart from his Alzheimer's disease, his eyesight is beginning to fail and he is starting to have difficulties walking because of arthritis.

Christopher has three children, Monica, Mark, and Amy. Mark and Amy live out of state, so the main care giving responsibilities fall on Christopher's oldest daughter Monica who lives in a nearby city. Monica drives to Glenview Village several times a week to see her father, usually spending half a day with him and taking care of needs around the apartment. Monica never complains, but Christopher worries that she is taking too much time away from her own husband and children in order to care for him. Christopher also worries about the high cost of his present and future care. He knows that people with Alzheimer's disease can still live for a long time, and his retirement "nest egg" really isn't all that much. He doesn't want his children to have to assume the cost of his care, especially with children of their own to educate.

Christopher dearly loves his six grandchildren, and much prizes the time he has spent with them since his retirement. He wants them to have good memories of their grandfather. He dreads the idea that they will eventually see him in a demented, debilitated state.

During the winter, Christopher suffers a mild stroke which leaves him with some difficulties with swallowing. For this reason, he is seeing Sarah Jones, a speech therapist.

During one therapy session, Christopher asks Sarah if she can help him make contact with Dr. Laura MacDonald. It is rumored around town that Dr. MacDonald has helped two elderly women commit suicide, and Sarah knows this. Sarah is suspicious of Christopher's intent and wonders how she should handle this situation.

■ ■ ■

The Legal Status of Physician Aid-in-Dying

In June 1997, the U.S. Supreme Court rendered a judgment in two cases concerning physician aid-in-dying, *Washington v. Glucksberg* and *Vacco v. Quill*. The Court "denied that assistance by physicians in suicide is a constitutionally protected right of terminally ill persons and their physicians" (3). At the same time, the Court did not completely rule out physician aid-in-dying, but put this question into the hands of the states. Six justices stated in their opinions that state legislatures remain the appropriate forum in which decriminalizing (and thus permitting) some kind of carefully controlled physician assistance in dying can be examined and, perhaps, experiments with it undertaken (3).

The first state to make physician aid-in-dying legal was Oregon which enacted the "Death with Dignity Act" on October 27, 1997. (4) In order to be eligible to participate in physician aid-in-dying under this Act, a patient must be:

- 18 years of age or older;
- a resident of Oregon;
- capable of making and communicating health care decisions for him/herself;
- diagnosed with a terminal illness that will lead to death within six months. (4)

Further, the following conditions must be met for an eligible patient to actually get a prescription for lethal medication from a physician:

- The patient must make two oral requests to the attending physician, separated by at least 15 days.
- The patient must provide a written request to the attending physician, signed in the presence of two witnesses, at least one of whom is not related to the patient.
- The attending physician and a consulting physician must confirm the patient's diagnosis and prognosis.
- The attending physician and a consulting physician must determine whether the patient is capable of making and communicating health care decisions for himself or herself.
- If either physician believes the patient's judgment is impaired by a psychiatric or psychological disorder (such as depression), the patient must be referred for a psychological examination.
- The attending physician must inform the patient of feasible alternatives to the Act including comfort care, hospice care, and pain control.
- The attending physician must request, but may not require, the patient to notify his her next-of-kin of the prescription request.
- A patient can rescind a request at any time and in any manner. The attending physician will also offer the patient an opportunity to rescind his or her request at the end of the 15-day waiting period following the initial request to participate (4).

Proponents of physician aid-in-dying would contend that these requirements serve to protect patients and to guard against abuses of the practice of physician aid-in-dying.

Other states which have legalized physician aid-in-dying have very similar stipulations in their laws (2).

If a patient lives in a state in which physician-aid-in-dying is not legal or if a patient does not qualify for this procedure under the stipulations of her state, another option is Voluntary Stopping of Eating and Drinking (VSED) (5). VSED represents an intentional decision on the part of the patient to stop drinking liquids and eating food for the specific purpose of causing her death (6). For most people, death occurs about 10 days after the initiation of VSED (7). VSED should not be confused with the dying patient who naturally loses interest in eating and drinking (8).

The Defense of Euthanasia and Physician Aid-in-Dying

What are the arguments that might be offered in support of acts of euthanasia and physician aid-in-dying? How do people try to justify it?

First, these practices are defended as acts of compassion in relieving suffering:

> Many advocates of euthanasia assert that there is a significant number of cases in which even the best medical technology cannot alleviate the physical pain of the terminally ill. Moreover, our technological advances have done little or nothing to help ameliorate the psychological fear and existential anxiety experienced by all at the approach of death, more acutely by some than others. Indeed, the fear of being trapped on life-support machinery is clearly a new and modern fear. These advocates claim that we act out of compassionate concern for our fellow humans when we end their pointless suffering at their own request. (9)

In the first case scenario, Ruth Jackson is in the final stages of the dying process. She is in constant pain, which is not being relieved by medication. She cannot sleep, and wishes for her death. Why not compassionately end her suffering now, as her husband wishes? After all, it is accepted practice to put animals out of their misery. Should we not be at least as kind to human beings? (10)

Another argument offered in favor of euthanasia and physician aid-in-dying is that these practices promote death with dignity. Human dignity "is violated, those who favor assisted suicide/euthanasia maintain, when we are forced to go through an agonizing period of pain and suffering before our lives end" (11). And "our dignity is assaulted, not only by physical pain, but by the depersonalization associated with prolonged use of life-sustaining technology, loss of control over our bodily functions, and the deterioration of our health . . ." (11). With euthanasia and assisted suicide, a patient can end his life when he is still "himself," and be remembered that way by his loved ones (10). In the second case scenario, Christopher Vaughn is becoming increasing debilitated physically (arthritis, failing eyesight, stroke). He faces increasing mental deterioration because of Alzheimer's disease. He dreads the idea that his grandchildren will see him in a demented and debilitated state.

Further, a value much emphasized in contemporary health care ethics is patient autonomy (see Chapter 1). But "if self-determination is a value, then it is important that each individual be allowed to control the manner, circumstances, and time of death" (9; see also 11). Christopher Vaughn is seeking physician aid-in-dying. Although he is in the early stages of Alzheimer's disease, he presumably still has the mental competency to make such a decision, and the principle of autonomy would say that he should have this option.

An analogy with the rightness of decisions to withdraw treatment has also been used to support euthanasia and physician aid-in-dying (11). Consider the following scenario:

> . . . two terminally ill people with the same condition, such as pancreatic cancer, both face a difficult period of dying. Should one suffer respiratory arrest, he could be put on a ventilator, which then could be withdrawn, allowing him to die. Another might not be fortunate enough to arrest. He would continue to live, experiencing pain and suffering until he dies. (11)

It is argued that "there is a lack of equity . . . between the way that these two patients are treated," and that this inequity could be remedied if euthanasia and physician aid-in-dying were made available to the latter (11). If Ruth Jackson were on a ventilator, removing it might be a way of allowing death to occur and ending her suffering. However, she does not have that option. Neither is Christopher Vaughn currently on any life-prolonging treatments that might be withdrawn to allow his death. Euthanasia and physician aid-in-dying would provide them with the same opportunity for death to occur as have patients who, through "the luck of the draw," are on life-sustaining treatments that can be stopped.

Finally, many believe that there are exceptions to the general prohibition against killing and that taking human life can sometimes be legitimate. Examples might be self-defense, the killing that takes place during a just war and, some would add, capital punishment. Some argue that this list should be expanded to include euthanasia and physician aid-in-dying for the terminally ill and for those suffering from irreversible, progressively debilitating diseases like multiple sclerosis or Alzheimer's (11). The justification for this expansion is utilitarian (see Chapter 1); namely, that the willful taking of life can be morally justified if the good desired outweighs the potential evil and that good cannot be achieved in a less destructive manner (11). In the case at hand, it is argued that "the greater value could be achieved in a person's life, *taken as a whole*, if he knew that at a certain stage of his dying he would be painlessly put to death rather than be allowed to linger on" (11).

Opposition to Euthanasia and Physician Aid-in-Dying

A theoretical argument against euthanasia and physician aid-in-dying comes from natural law ethics. Basically, this theory maintains that an action which is in accord with human nature is right while an action which goes against human nature is wrong (see Chapter 1). Euthanasia (and physician aid-in-dying) are seen as going against the natural human inclination for self-preservation, and therefore are judged morally wrong:

> Every human being has a natural inclination to continue living. Our reflexes and responses fit us to fight against attackers, flee wild animals, and dodge out of the way of trucks. In our daily lives we exercise the caution and care necessary to protect ourselves. Our bodies are similarly structured for survival right down to the molecular level. When we are cut, our capillaries seal shut, our blood clots, and fibrinogen is produced to start the process of healing the wound. When we are invaded by bacteria, antibodies are produced to fight against the alien organisms, and their remains are swept out of the body by special cells designed for clean-up work . . . .
>
> It is enough, I believe, to recognize that the organization of the human body and our patterns of behavioral responses make the continuation of life a natural goal. By reason alone, then, we can recognize that euthanasia sets us against our own nature. (12)

Arguments of a more pragmatic character are also advanced against euthanasia and physician aid-in-dying. Thus it has been pointed out that medical diagnoses and prognoses can be mistaken. We all know of people who were told they had a short life expectancy because of a disease, and then unexpectedly recovered or substantially outlived the projections for how much time they had left. In particular, states allowing physician aid-in-dying may have a requirement that the patient have 6 months or less to live in order to be eligible for this procedure. However, data already collected suggest that a significant number of patients live beyond their 6-month prognosis (13). In sum, since medical diagnoses and prognoses are not 100 percent sure, the concern is that, if euthanasia and physician aid-in-dying are allowed, some people may end their lives needlessly or prematurely.

There is evidence that psychological factors are strong motivations for patients to request euthanasia or physician aid-in-dying. Patients themselves report that "the primary motive is not to escape physical pain but psychological distress" with the main drivers being "depression, hopelessness and fear of loss of autonomy and control" (14). However, "our response to suicidal feelings associated with depression and hopeless is not to give people the means to end their lives but to offer them counseling and caring" (14).

Further, there is concern that patients who are difficult or expensive to take care of may feel pressured by other people into opting for euthanasia or physician aid-in-dying when they really do not want this:

> Will we not sweep up, in the process, some who are not really tired of life, but think others are tired of them; some who do not really want to die, but who feel they should not live on, because to do so when there looms the legal alternative of euthanasia is to do a selfish or cowardly act? Will not some feel an obligation to have themselves "eliminated" in order that funds allocated for their terminal care might be better used by their families or, financial worries aside, in order to relieve their families of the emotional strain involved? (15)

For example, Christopher Vaughn's oldest daughter Monica drives from a nearby city several times a week to see him, usually spending half a day with him and taking care of needs around the apartment. Christopher worries that she is taking too much time away from her own husband and children in order to care for him. He also worries about the high cost of his present and future care since he knows that people with Alzheimer's disease can live for a long time. His retirement "nest egg" really isn't all that much, and he doesn't want his children to have to assume the cost of his care, especially with children of their own to educate. Altogether, these are subtle pressures that may be pushing Christopher to consider physician aid-in-dying.

Further, there is fear that a slippery slope effect will occur. In other words, there is fear that if we allow euthanasia and physician aid-in-dying in some cases, the practice might expand to include other cases in which these practices are highly questionable. For example, we might start out with voluntary euthanasia and physician aid-in-dying, wherein life is ended at the request of the patient. But this might expand to cases of involuntary euthanasia in which someone other than the patient decides that a patient's life is to be ended:

> . . . if the warrant for assisted suicide/euthanasia is to relieve suffering, there is no reason why these practices should be limited to those who are competent. Why not provide killing for those who are suffering and can no longer speak for themselves? If suffering provides a moral warrant for voluntary euthanasia, it should also provide a warrant for nonvoluntary euthanasia. (11)

Indeed, "the experience of the Netherlands shows that nonvoluntary euthanasia can follow voluntary euthanasia, even when this is not planned" (11). Or, we might start out with allowing euthanasia and physician aid-in-dying for those who are terminally ill and find it expanding to the chronically ill and incurable, and even to those with psychiatric disorders (11). In the case of Dr. Jack Kevorkian, a Michigan physician who openly practiced aid-in-dying, the practice extended to a person whose condition was not life-threatening and may well have been treatable. The 35th person he helped commit suicide was Judith Curren, a woman suffering from chronic fatigue syndrome, a weight problem, and depression (16).

The impact of euthanasia and physician aid-in-dying on health care providers and services has also been an issue. Fundamentally, persons in the health care professions are healers. It is feared that combining killing with healing would result in confusion and distrust of health care providers among patients, and undermine the relationship of health care providers with their patients (11). Further, in the era of managed care and cost containment, euthanasia and physician aid-in-dying could come to "be seen as cheaper alternatives for health care systems than palliative care for the dying or ameliorative treatment for the incurable" (11). Indeed, "in a social context where medical care is already limited according to race, gender, and ability to pay, a policy of euthanasia might be implemented more readily for the poor, racial minorities, and women than for others" (11).

Finally, it has been pointed out that "many things can go wrong during an assisted suicide" (14). Patients can vomit up the pills they take, or may not take enough pills, or may wake up instead of dying (14). For example, patients in a Dutch study "vomited up their medications in 7 percent of cases; in 15 percent of cases, patients either did not die or took a very long time to die—hours, even days; in 18 percent, doctors had to intervene to administer a lethal medication themselves, converting a physician-assisted suicide into euthanasia" (14). In sum, the procedure of physician aid-in-dying may not succeed in achieving its goal of a "good death" for a patient (14).

Managing Pain and Relieving Suffering

Some opponents of euthanasia and physician aid-in-dying have campaigned for better palliative care for the dying (3). Recognizing that a cure cannot be achieved, palliative care aims at "pain and symptom relief and the care of the patient as a whole person and as a social being during the experience of illness" (8). Palliative care "includes but is not limited to hospice care and comfort care near death" (8). As one proponent of palliative care states, ". . . people involved in health care have now what may be a brief window of opportunity to increase their efforts to improve and refine palliative medicine and hospice practice so that fewer and fewer persons imagine that PAD [physician-assisted dying] is their only hope, as they live in fear of unrelieved suffering and indignity in their dying as a consequence of medical neglect" (3).

Various factors can be barriers to good pain management. One factor is a lack of training of health care workers in good pain management techniques. Some health care workers do not know what is available for pain management and how to use it effectively (17). This may be true in the case of Ruth Jackson. Due to her cancer, Ruth is described as suffering intense pain, but "studies indicate that as many as 95 percent" of cancer patients "*can* get good pain relief if skilled practitioners administer the right medications in the right ways" (17).

Another factor that can negatively impact good pain management is fear of the patient becoming addicted to the pain medication (18, 19). However, a distinction can be made between *addiction* and *drug dependence.* In the case of drug dependency, the drug has a medical value for the person taking it. The dependency is a physical, rather than a psychological, problem. Withdrawal symptoms will occur if the drug is taken away suddenly, so that the drug needs to be withdrawn gradually, over a period of time. Addiction, on the other hand, is a psychological problem. The drug has no medical value for the person taking it, but the individual desires it and is driven to obtain it (19, 20).

If Ruth Jackson had been given pain medication in doses sufficient to control her severe pain, she may well have become physically dependent on it, but this does not mean that she should be considered an addict. Moreover, in the case of someone who is dying, like Ruth Jackson, the pain medication need never be stopped to cause withdrawal symptoms (20).

Other cultural factors may also hinder good pain management. In the minds of some people the term "narcotic" (i.e., opioid) automatically evokes an image of street drugs (19). Unfortunately, the stigma attached to narcotics may carry over into the health care setting, where such drugs have perfectly legitimate uses (21).

From an ethical point of view, the classic question about pain management at the end of life has concerned the use of medications that may hasten death. Specifically, there has been concern about narcotics depressing respiration and, in this way, having a secondary effect of hastening the patient's death. Such a secondary effect has made some health care providers hesitant about administering these pain medications for fear that they are engaging in an act of euthanasia (20, 22). These concerns might well arise in a case like that of Ruth Jackson, where high doses of opioids would likely be needed to control her severe cancer pain.

Traditionally, the answer has been that it is ethically permissible to use medications to relieve pain that may have a side effect of hastening the time of death based on the *principle of double effect* (17, 18). This ethical principle applies to situations in which a single action will have two different consequences. One of the consequences is perfectly good and is what is intended. The second consequence, however, is bad and is not really wanted, but it comes along as a side effect of the action. The principle of double effect says that it is ethically permissible to take an action with such double consequences. More exactly, the principle of double effect can be stated as follows:

> This doctrine, which is designed to provide moral guidance for an action that could have at least one bad and one good effect, holds that such an action is permissible if it satisfies these four conditions: (1) The act itself must be morally good or neutral (for example, administering a pain-killer); (2) only the good consequences of the action must be intended (relief of the patient's suffering); (3) the good effect must not be produced by means of the evil effect (the relief of suffering must not be produced by the patient's death); (4) there must be some weighty reason for permitting the evil (the relief of great suffering, which can only be achieved through a high risk of death). (22)

Intent is critical in using the principle of double effect. It must be pain relief, not the patient's death, that is intended in administering the medication. But how does one know someone's intent in administering pain medication? This is one way: if a patient's pain is relieved by a certain dosage level of the pain medication, the level will not be deliberately increased to risk depression of respiration (and death). This indicates that the intent is indeed to relieve pain.

Fortunately, this ethical concern about pain medication is becoming outdated. First of all, "there is some evidence that administering narcotic agents in amounts sufficient to provide adequate pain relief may extend, rather than shorten, life" (20). This is so because "patients without pain are more likely to accept a greater degree of nourishment, to be more active and less depressed, and to be more open to other treatment possibilities," and, "as a result, they may live longer" (20). Second, more is now known about how to administer pain medication in a way that avoids depression of respiration:

> Health care professionals who are accustomed to giving one to two milligrams of morphine in the emergency room or coronary care unit for the relief of moderate acute pain need to know that some patients may need, and can tolerate, 1,000 milligrams or more of morphine per hour,

as in intravenous infusion, to control the ferocious pain of some cancers. Such doses are not reached overnight but infusions are judiciously titrated upwards in measured increments until pain is contained. In this way respiratory distress does not occur, since unrelieved pain acts as a physiological antagonist to the respiratory depressant effect of the opiate drug. (23)

Finally, it is now recognized that respiratory depression and arrest is a normal part of the dying process, and we need to be careful not to falsely see it as caused by pain medication:

> However, current medical research raises questions about the need to apply the principle of double effect to pain management. As the chair of the Wisconsin Cancer Pain Initiative stated in correspondence to the Council of Ethical and Judicial Affairs of the American Medical Association, "Death from respiratory depression is exceedingly rare in patients with cancer who chronically receive opioid analgesics for pain. As a person nears death, there is deterioration in respiratory function. However, these respiratory changes should not be confused with the effects of opioids. (18)

In sum, there is no reason to withhold adequate doses of pain medication from dying patients for fear of hastening their deaths.

It has been estimated that "between 5% and 35% of hospice patients have intractable symptoms in the last week of life" which may include "pain, shortness of breath, dyspnea, nausea and vomiting" (24). In such cases a procedure known as *palliative sedation* may be used.

Palliative sedation "refers to the use of sedating medications to relieve refractory and intolerable symptoms, such as pain, dyspnea, and agitated delirium, after all other measures have failed" (8). In particular, "a reduction in the patient's level of consciousness is anticipated and accepted as a necessary part of this therapy" (8); indeed, the patient "may require sedation to unconsciousness" (8).

The American Medical Association has taken the position that the use of palliative sedation to the point of unconsciousness is ethically permissible under certain conditions, including:

- The patient is in the final stages of terminal illness.
- The patient's clinical symptoms have been unresponsive to aggressive, symptom-specific treatments.

■ There has been consultation with an interdisciplinary team, if available, including an expert in the field of palliative care, to ensure that symptom-specific treatments have been sufficiently employed.

■ The patient and/or the patient's surrogate have given informed consent for palliative sedation to unconsciousness.

■ Palliative sedation is not being used to intentionally cause the patient's death (25).

The American Medical Association adds the qualification that "palliative sedation is not an appropriate response to suffering that is primarily existential," that is, "the experience of agony and distress that may arise from such issues as death anxiety, isolation and loss of control" (25). By way of example, "palliative sedation is not the way to address suffering created by social isolation and loneliness" (25); rather, "such suffering should be addressed by providing the patient with needed social support" (25).

In the case study at the beginning of this chapter, palliative sedation to unconsciousness might be an option in the case of Ruth Jackson. Indeed, this procedure has been proposed as an alternative to the practices of euthanasia and physician aid-in-dying. While acknowledging that "a brief life of nearly continuous sedation is not of great merit," it is argued that "continuous sedation achieves a humane and compassionate period of dying for patient, caregivers, and family without precipitating the very serious concerns about 'slippery slopes' that arise with acceptance of direct killing" (26).

While we have been focusing on the management of physical pain and symptoms, it is important to keep in mind that the suffering that accompanies the dying process goes beyond the physical. Providing emotional and psychological support for those who are ill is likewise part of good care of the dying. As one church document states:

> The pleas of gravely ill people who sometimes ask for death are . . . almost always a case of an anguished plea for help and love. What a sick person needs, besides medical care, is love, the human and supernatural warmth with which the sick person can and ought to be surrounded by all those close to him or her, parents and children, doctors and nurses. (27)
>
> As for those who work in the medical profession, they ought to neglect no means of making all their skill available to the sick and the dying; but they should also remember how much more necessary it is to provide them with the comfort of boundless kindness and heartfelt charity (27).

CHAPTER SUMMARY

Key Terms and Concepts

euthanasia: a person other than the patient intentionally performs an act that is the direct, immediate cause of the patient's death.

voluntary euthanasia: an act of euthanasia undertaken at the request of or with the consent of the patient.

involuntary euthanasia: an act of euthanasia undertaken without the consent of the patient.

physician aid-in-dying: a physician provides a patient with the means (typically drugs) to cause his or her own death.

principle of double effect: it is ethically permissible to take a course of action that has an evil effect accompanying a good one provided that the act itself is ethically good or neutral, only the good consequence of the action is intended, the good effect is not produced by means of the evil effect, and there is some weighty reason for permitting the evil.

palliative sedation: the use of sedating medications to relieve refractory and intolerable symptoms.

Key Points

- Physician aid-in-dying (although not euthanasia) has been legalized in several states. The practice is governed by specific requirements.
- Arguments given *in support of* euthanasia and physician aid-in-dying include the following:
  * Euthanasia and physician aid-in-dying are acts of compassion in relieving suffering.
  * Euthanasia and physician aid-in-dying promote death with dignity.
  * Choosing the time of one's death is an exercise of autonomy.
  * Euthanasia and physician aid-in-dying provide the same opportunity for death that is available to patients able to have life-sustaining treatments withdrawn.
  * We already recognize some cases in which it is legitimate to take human life, and euthanasia and physician aid-in-dying should be included.

- Arguments *against* euthanasia and physician aid-in-dying include the following:
  * These practices violate natural law ethics in going against the natural human inclination for self-preservation.
  * If euthanasia and physician aid-in-dying are allowed, some patients may end their lives needlessly or prematurely because medical diagnoses and prognoses can be mistaken.
  * Psychological factors, such as depression, hopelessness and fear of loss of autonomy and control, are strong motivations for patients to request euthanasia or physician aid-in-dying so that these patients should be offered counseling, not death.
  * Patients could feel pressured to end their lives by financial considerations or in order to relieve significant others of the strains of care giving.
  * Allowing euthanasia and physician aid-in-dying in the case of terminally ill patients by their request or with their consent could have a slippery slope effect, leading to involuntary euthanasia and even to ending the lives of patients whose conditions are not life threatening and may be treatable.
  * Euthanasia and physician aid-in-dying are incompatible with the traditional role of health care workers as healers, and could lead to a decline in the quality of medical care made available to debilitated and dying patients.
  * The procedures used in physician aid-in-dying may not succeed as intended in bringing about an easy death for the patient.
- Lack of training of health care workers in pain management, the fear of addiction, and the association of narcotic medications with street drugs can all be barriers to good pain management.
- The classic ethical question about pain management at the end of life has been the use of medications that may hasten death. According to the principle of double effect, it is ethically permissible to use sufficient medication to control pain although that medication has a side effect of hastening a patient's death. However, the possibility of this side effect of pain medication occurring has become largely outdated.
- In the case of a patient in the final stages of terminal illness suffering from severe pain or other distressing physical symptoms which cannot be relieved, palliative sedation to unconsciousness may be an alternative to euthanasia or physician aid-in-dying.

FOR FURTHER DISCUSSION

1. In your judgment, what are the three strongest arguments offered *in favor of* euthanasia and physician aid-in-dying? Why do you find the other arguments less strong or implausible?

2. In your judgment, what are the three strongest arguments offered *against* euthanasia and physician aid-in-dying? Why do you find the other arguments less strong or implausible?

3. Suppose that the legalization of physician aid-in-dying was placed on the ballot in your state. How would you vote, and why?

4. In our first case scenario, Tom Jackson asks physician assistant Mark Bennett to euthanize his wife. Suppose you were Mark Bennett. How do you think you would react to this situation? What would you say to Tom? What courses of action might be options for handling this situation?

5. In our second case scenario, Christopher Vaughn essentially asks speech therapist Sarah Jones to help him arrange physician aid-in-dying. Suppose you were Sarah Jones. How do you think you would react to this situation? What would you say to Christopher? What courses of action might be options for handling this situation?

6. If you are a member of a faith community, research your faith community's views on euthanasia and physician aid-in-dying. Then compare in class the positions and statements of the various religious groups. (Keep in mind that you may be caring for patients whose decisions on death and dying issues will be guided by the position of their religious group.)

References

1. Sydney Leach, "*Europe's Increasing Acceptance of Euthanasia and Assisted Suicide.*" Accessed April 2016. http://www.nationalreview.com/article/398521/europes-increasing-acceptance-euthanasia-and-assisted-suicide-sydney-leach.

2. ProCon.org, "*State-by-State Guide to Physician-Assisted Suicide.*" http://euthanasia.procon.org/view.resource.php?resourceID=000132. Accessed April 2016.

3. James F. Bresnahan, "Palliative Care or Assisted Suicide?" *America* (1998): 16–21.

4. Oregon Public Health Division, *FAQs About the Death With Dignity Act.* http://healthoregon.org/dwd. Accessed April 2016.

5. Neil Lake, "*Aid-In-Dying Loophole: Advocates Want You to Know You Can Stop Eating and Drinking.*" http://commonhealth.wbur.org/2014/04/dying-loophole-stop-eating-and-drinking. Accessed April 2016.

6. Patients Rights Council, "*Voluntarily Stopping Eating & Drinking Important Questions and Answers.*" http://www.patientsrightscouncil.org/site/wp-content/uploads/2013/03/VSED_Questions.pdf. Accessed April 2016.

7. Death With Dignity, "*Other Options to Hasten Your Death.*" https://www.deathwithdignity.org/options-to-hasten-death. Accessed April 2016.

8. Nancy Berlinger, Bruce Jennings, and Susan M. Wolf, *The Hastings Center Guidelines for Decisions on Life-Sustaining Treatment and Care Near the End of Life: Revised. and Expanded Second Edition* (New York, NY: Oxford University Press, 2013).

9. Michael Manning, *Euthanasia and Physician-Assisted Suicide Killing or Caring?* (New York/Mahwah, NJ: Paulist Press, 1998).

10. "Help Me Die," Fanlight Productions, DVD.

11. Committee on Medical Ethics of the Episcopal Diocese of Washington, DC, *Assisted Suicide and Euthanasia Christian Moral Perspectives* (Harrisburg, PA: Morehouse Publishing, 1997).

12. J. Gay-Williams, "The Wrongfulness of Euthanasia" in *Intervention and Reflection: Basic Issues in Medical Ethics,* ed. Ronald Munson (Belmont, CA: Thomson Wadsworth, 2008).

13. Herbert Hendin and Kathleen Foley, "*Physician-Assisted Suicide in Oregon: A Medical Perspective,*" http://dredf.org/assisted_suicide/HendinFoley_MichiganLawReview.pdf. Accessed April 2016.

14. Ezekiel J. Emanuel, "*Four Myths About Doctor-Assisted Suicide,*" http://opinionator.blogs.nytimes.com/2012/10/27/four-myths-about-doctor-assisted-suicide. Accessed April 2016.

15. Yale Kamisar, "From Euthanasia Legislation: Some Non-Religious Objections" in *Euthanasia and the Right to Die,* ed. A.B. Downing (New York, NY: Humanities Press, 1970).

16. Chicago Tribune, "Kevorkian Steps Over a Fine Line," reprinted in the (Dubuque) *Telegraph-Herald,* August 23, 1996.

17. Phebe Saunders Haugen, "Pain Relief: Legal Aspects of Pain Relief for the Dying," *Minnesota Medicine* 80 (November 1997): 15–18.

18. Thomas E. Elliott, "Pain Control at the End of Life," *Minnesota Medicine* 80 (November 1997): 27–32.

19. "Quality of Mercy: A Case for Better Pain Management," produced by Richard J. Adler, Filmmakers Library. Videocassette.

20. Hastings Center, *Guidelines on the Termination of Life-Sustaining Treatment and the Care of the Dying* (Briarcliff Manor, NY: Hastings Center, 1987).

21. Russell K. Portenoy, Vincent Dole, Herman Joseph, Joyce Lowinson, Carolyn Rice, Sharon Segal, and Beverly L. Richman, "Pain Management and Chemical Dependency," *Journal of the American Medical Association* 278/7 (August 20, 1997): 592–93.

22. President's Commission for the Study of Ethical Problems in Medicine and Biomedical and Behavioral Research, *Deciding to Forego Life-Sustaining Treatment* (New York, NY: Concern for Dying, 1983; reprint).

23. Catholic Health Association of the United States, *Care of the Dying* (St. Louis, MO: Catholic Health Association of the United States, 1993).

24. Kevin B. O'Reilly, "*AMA Meeting: AMA OKs Palliative Sedation for Terminally Ill,*" http://www.ama-assn.org/amed-news/2008/07/07/prsi0707. Accessed January 2009.

25. American Medical Association, "*Opinion 2.201—Sedation to Unconsciousness in End-of-Life Care.*" http://www.ama-assn.org/ama/pub/physician-resources /medical-ethics/code-medical-ethics/opinion2201.page? Accessed April 2016.

26. Joanne Lynn, "Morpheus or Death: The Case of Nicholas Miklovick" in *Casebook on the Termination of Life-Sustaining Treatment and the Care of the Dying,* ed. Cynthia B. Cohen (Bloomington, IN: Indiana University Press, 1988).

27. Vatican Congregation for the Doctrine of the Faith, *Declaration on Euthanasia* (Washington, DC: United States Catholic Conference, 1980).

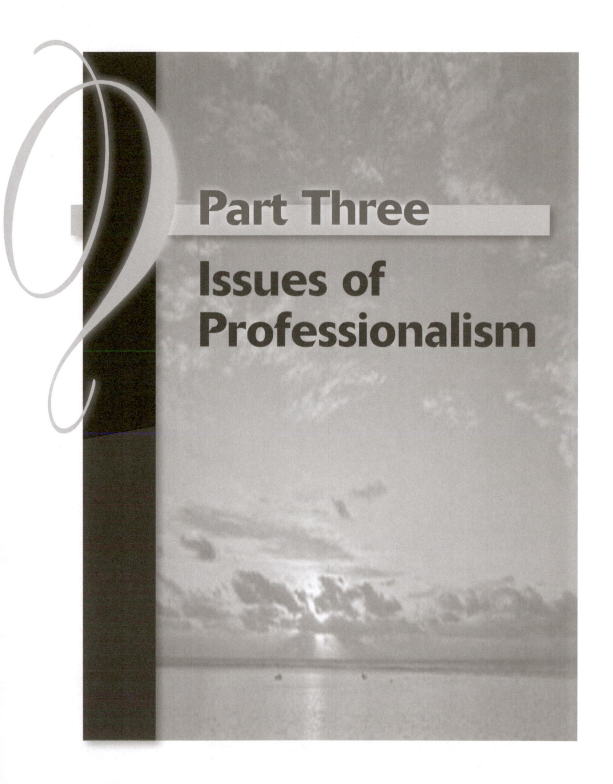

Part Three

Issues of Professionalism

Chapter 12

Confidentiality

Leaks of supposedly confidential or privileged information to the media have become commonplace in American society. Such leaks are a way of life. This attitude makes it harder to appreciate why confidentiality is emphasized and expected in health care. Yet confidentiality goes back to the Hippocratic oath: "Whatever I see or hear, professionally or privately, which ought not be divulged, I will keep secret and tell no one" (1)

In this chapter you will learn about:

- The reasons why confidentiality is an important value in health care;
- The ethical principle governing confidentiality;
- When it is ethically legitimate to break confidentiality;
- Some challenges to maintaining confidentiality;
- Governmental regulations pertaining to confidentiality in health care.

Case Study

Eleanor Murray works in the medical records department at Lakeland Hospital. One day her supervisor asks her to review some medical records to check on insurance claims for a particular company. One of the files she is supposed to review belongs to Roger Faber. In looking through the file, Eleanor notices that Roger has undergone testing for the gene for Huntington's disease because of a history of this disease in his family, and has tested positive. Huntington's disease affects persons during their adult years, and involves worsening gait, constant uncontrollable movement, and personality changes. Death usually comes ten to fifteen years after the onset of symptoms. If someone has the gene for Huntington's disease, it is almost inevitable that he will eventually be affected by the disease.

This discovery upsets Eleanor very much since her sister Jean is engaged to marry Roger. Does her sister know about Roger's genetic status? How will this affect their marriage? Should Jean be burdened with heavy caregiving responsibilities for Roger? Will Jean have to forgo having her own biological children to prevent Huntington's disease from being passed on to them?

Eleanor has always been protective of her sister Jean. Eleanor knows that any information she sees in medical records is supposed to be kept confidential. At the same time, she doesn't want to see her sister get hurt. She struggles with the question of whether she should break confidentiality and tell Jean about Roger's genetic status.

■ ■ ■

Why Confidentiality Is a Value in Health Care

There are several justifications for maintaining confidentiality in health care practice. Based on the ethical principle of autonomy (see Chapter 1), an individual has a right to control personal information and to protect privacy (2). A health care professional would not "show proper respect for the patient's autonomy and privacy if he or she does not uphold the confidentiality of the professional–patient relationship" (3). Consequentialist ethics (see Chapter 1) also provides an underpinning for confidentiality (3, 4). For "if patients could not trust physicians to conceal some information from third parties, patients would be reluctant to disclose full and forthright information or to authorize a complete examination and a full battery of tests" (4). And, "without such information, physicians would not be able to make accurate diagnoses and prognoses or to recommend the best course of treatment" (4). The concern that, without assurance of confidentiality, patients may not disclose all relevant information to health care providers or be deterred from seeking treatment altogether is reinforced by the fact that some medical problems are quite personal, such as infertility and sexually transmitted diseases. It is also reinforced by the fact that some diseases, such as acquired immunodeficiency syndrome (AIDS) and mental illness, have carried a social stigma and may lead to discrimination (2, 5).

To appreciate the value of confidentiality, just consider what appears on the evening news when the President of the United States or another prominent person has a serious health problem and must have surgery or other treatment. Would you want this kind of information broadcast about yourself?

The Principle of Confidentiality

As an ethical principle, *there is a strong prima facie obligation to maintain confidentiality about a patient's health information* (4). In others words, there is an expectation that confidentiality be maintained about someone's health information, unless the value of maintaining confidentiality is overridden by exceptional circumstances. The exceptional circumstances that are recognized to justify breaking confidentiality are *substantial threats to others, to the public interest, or to the patient* (4).

The ethical theories that support maintaining confidentiality also allow for exceptions to the rule. The ethical theory of principlism (see Chapter 1) recognizes the principle of nonmaleficence (the duty to avoid harm) as well as the principle of autonomy (which supports an individual's right to control personal information), with nonmaleficence sometimes limiting and taking precedence over autonomy (2). Consequentialist ethics (see Chapter 1) requires that "we compare the benefits of keeping confidences with the benefits of revealing confidential information in circumstances in which the information is desperately needed by another party" (3). And "if through this comparison it turns out that there is an overriding duty to warn persons who might be seriously harmed if confidentiality were maintained, then confidentiality is not an absolute duty" (3).

In some cases, breaking confidentiality may be considered ethically *permissible*. In other cases, an argument might be made that it is morally *obligatory* to do so; for example, when there is a high probability of some major harm coming to a person other than the patient (4).

What are examples of cases in which breaking confidentiality would be considered legitimate from an ethical point of view? One example involves the transmission of HIV/AIDS to another person, and hence, the transmission of a potentially fatal disease:

> In one case, after several weeks of dry persistent coughing and night sweats, a bisexual man visited his family physician, who arranged for a test to determine whether he had antibodies to HIV. The physician informed the patient of a positive test, of the risk of infection for his wife, and of the risk that their children might lose both parents. The patient refused to tell his wife and insisted that the physician maintain absolute confidentiality. The physician reluctantly yielded to this demand. Only in the last few weeks of his life did the patient allow the physician to inform his wife of the nature of the husband's illness, and a test then showed that she too was antibody-positive for HIV. When symptoms appeared a year later, she angrily, and we think appropriately, accused the physician of violating his moral responsibilities to her and to her children. This case presents a high probability (if we assume unprotected sexual intercourse) of a major harm to an identifiable individual—the paradigm case of a justified breach of confidentiality. (4)

Or again, breaking confidentiality may be necessary in the case of involuntary commitment proceedings for a patient who is apt to commit suicide or engage in self-mutilating behavior. This breach of confidentiality falls into the category of preventing serious harm to the patient himself. Legally, health care workers may be required to report cases of child abuse, gunshot wounds, and cases of contagious diseases (4).

However, it should be emphasized that such breaches of confidentiality are *exceptional cases*. Apart from legally mandated reporting requirements, health care workers should be extremely cautious about breaking confidentiality. It should always be a "last resort," after alternative courses of action have been explored and failed (4).

Challenges to Maintaining Confidentiality

There has been increasing sensitivity to potential breaches of confidentiality in the workplace setting, ranging from casual conversations about patients in the elevator and cafeteria to misdialing fax machines to computer screens being left in a position visible to anyone walking by. Health care workers are being educated on avoiding such breaches of confidentiality.

However, challenges to maintaining confidentiality about patient information extend beyond the workplace setting. For example, "it isn't unusual for people to talk about their workplace with a spouse, family member, and friends" (6). In fact, "one of the first questions that greets many of us as we walk through the door at the end of each workday is, 'How was your day?'" (6). But "the problem for health care providers is that discussions about the workplace have the potential to jeopardize patient confidentiality" (6). While "confidentiality training in health care facilities discusses the need for discretion in the workplace," it often "fails to address how to handle requests for information that come from friends, family, and neighbors" (6).

Living in a small community "where everybody knows everybody else" poses a special challenge to maintaining confidentiality about health information. A patient may find a member of her church or a neighbor, or even a cousin or relative by marriage, among the staff working at the local medical clinic where she seeks care.

Yet another challenge to be met is the large number of health care workers involved in the care of a particular patient who can (and need to) have access to his medical records:

A patient of mine with mild chronic obstructive pulmonary disease was transferred from the surgical intensive-care unit to a surgical nursing floor two days after an elective cholecystectomy. On the day of the transfer, the patient saw a respiratory therapist writing in his medical chart . . . and became concerned about the confidentiality of his hospital records. The patient threatened to leave the hospital prematurely unless I could guarantee that the confidentiality of his hospital record would be respected.

The patient's complaint prompted me to enumerate the number of persons who had both access to his hospital record and a reason to examine it. I was amazed to learn that at least 25 and possibly as many as 100 health professionals and administrative personnel at our university hospital had access to the patient's record. . . . These persons included 6 attending physicians (the primary physician, the surgeon, the pulmonary consultant, and others); 12 house officers (medical, surgical, intensive-care unit, and "covering" house staff); 20 nursing personnel (on three shifts); 6 respiratory therapists; 3 nutritionists; 2 clinical pharmacists; 15 students (from medicine, nursing, respiratory therapy, and clinical pharmacy); 4 unit secretaries; 4 hospital financial officers; and 4 chart reviewers (utilization review, quality assurance review, tissue review, and insurance auditor).

> . . . I suggested to the patient that these people were all involved in providing or supporting his health-care services. . . . Despite my reassurances the patient was obviously distressed and retorted, "I always believed that medical confidentiality was part of a doctor's code of ethics. Perhaps you should tell me just what you people mean by 'confidentiality'!" (7)

One way of responding to this problem is for health care facilities and services to emphasize confidentiality as a job expectation of everyone involved in patient care, whether directly or indirectly, and no matter what his or her particular job is. In fact, it has been suggested that job descriptions for health care workers should explicitly mention respect for confidentiality among job qualifications, that all employees who have access to patient information should be asked to sign a confidentiality agreement annually, and that one standard by which a health care worker's job performance should be evaluated is his demonstrated respect for patient confidentiality (8).

HIPAA Regulations

In 1996, the U.S. Congress enacted the Health Insurance Portability and Accountability Act (HIPAA). In addition to requirements concerning the transferability of health insurance, this legislation provides a comprehensive framework for regulating the standardization, security, and privacy of health information. The HIPAA statute as such focuses on the electronic exchange of health information. However, as implemented by the U.S. Department of Health and Human Services, HIPAA regulations are much broader and govern essentially all collection, maintenance, transmission, use, and disclosure of "individually identifiable health information." The regulations address standards for transactions (such as health claims and health care payments) to enable the electronic interchange of health information, for a unique health identifier for each individual, for code sets for appropriate data elements for transactions, for security of health information, for electronic signatures, for transfer of information among health plans, and for privacy (9). The privacy standards in particular interface with the ethical issue of confidentiality.

The Privacy Rule mandates that health care facilities and services have in place privacy policies and procedures appropriate for their services, notify patients about their privacy rights, and how their information can be used or disclosed, train employees in understanding the privacy practices, appoint a privacy official responsible for seeing that the privacy policies and procedures are implemented, and safeguard patients' records. (10)

HIPAA was reinforced by the Health Information Technology for Economic and Clinical Health Act (HITECH Act) of 2009. The HITECH Act provides for more rigorous enforcement of HIPAA through substantial mandatory financial penalties for "willful neglect," required audits of entities covered under the act, and notification of patients of any unsecured data breaches related to protected health information. (11)

Because allied health professionals handle patient medical records and requests for information from these records, they need to be informed about HIPAA regulations regarding what information can be released about patients' conditions and treatments. (10) Basically, HIPAA allows the use and disclosure of individually identifiable health information for purposes of treatment, payment, and health care operations; all other cases of use or disclosure of such information require a specific authorization by the patient (10).

To be compliant with HIPAA, a host of daily practices and procedures within a health care facility must be addressed. Do health care workers ever discuss patients among themselves or with family members in public areas of the facility? Do phone conversations occur in an area where patient information can be overheard? Are computer monitors positioned in such a way that unauthorized persons can see information about patients? Are fax machines monitored to ensure that material with patient information is not left available to unauthorized personnel? Are documents with patient information turned face down to avoid observation by visitors? (10). At first glance, such concerns may seem unwarrantedly detailed, onerous, and just another example of governmental bureaucracy. From a more positive perspective, they can be viewed as raising our consciousness about the many arenas in which the concept of confidentiality has applicability.

CHAPTER SUMMARY

Key Terms and Concepts

principle of confidentiality: a strong prima facie obligation exists to maintain confidentiality about a patient's health information. This obligation can be overridden by substantial threats to others, to the public interest, or to the patient.

HIPAA (Health Insurance Portability and Accountability Act): federal legislation that includes mandatory protections for individually identifiable health information.

Key Points

- Confidentiality is important in health care because, if it is not maintained, patients may be deterred from seeking treatment they need or may not want to disclose all the information necessary for effective treatment.
- Ethically, there is an expectation that health care professionals maintain confidentiality about the health information of patients to which they have access. The cases in which breaking confidentiality may be judged ethically permissible or even obligatory are the exception rather than the rule.
- Challenges to maintaining confidentiality can occur both within and outside of the workplace setting.
- Governmental regulations established by HIPAA have reinforced confidentiality in health care and spelled out concretely how it should be put into practice.

FOR FURTHER DISCUSSION

1. Consider the case of Eleanor Murray at the beginning of this chapter. Through her work in the medical records department of a hospital she has learned that Roger Faber, the fiancé of her sister Jean, has tested positive for Huntington's disease. She is debating whether she should break confidentiality and convey this information to her sister.

   - *Eleanor has to weigh the pros and cons of breaking confidentiality in this situation. What are the pros? The cons?*
   - *Role play a conversation between Eleanor and Jean in which Eleanor has decided to break confidentiality and to tell Jean about Roger's genetic status. What might be Jean's reaction if this information is news to her? On the other hand, what might be Jean's reaction if she already knows about Roger's genetic status?*
   - *Considering the ethical principle governing confidentiality, is it justifiable for Eleanor to break confidentiality? Are there any relevant differences between this situation and the case of HIV/AIDS presented in the chapter as a "paradigm case of a justified breach of confidentiality"?*
   - *Considering HIPAA regulations, is it legally permissible for Eleanor to break confidentiality?*
   - *Eleanor is genuinely concerned about the future welfare of her sister. Is there any way Eleanor can handle this situation without breaking confidentiality about the medical record she has seen?*

2. St. Margaret's Hospital is located in a small, rural community. The population of the town is 5,000, and it is surrounded by farms. It is a community that prides itself on being "neighborly."

   Jerry Johnson is a physical therapist at St. Margaret's. While he is shopping in the grocery store one evening, an elderly neighbor, Mrs. Todd, stops to talk with him. Mrs. Todd knows that a little boy down the street from her was hospitalized yesterday after being hit by a car. She asks Jerry if he knows how this little boy is doing.

   Jerry has been giving treatments to the little boy since he arrived at the hospital. Without thinking, Jerry gives Mrs. Todd a fairly detailed report on the boy's injuries and the progress he is making toward recovery. After all, she seems as concerned about him as if he were her own grandchild!

   Jerry broke confidentiality by sharing medical information about the injured boy with his neighbor. Clearly, this breach was neither ethically justified nor legally permissible. It is all too easy for health care workers to break confidentiality in casual conversations without thinking. What kind of responses might health care workers prepare to have ready in these kinds of situations?

3. At Oaklawn Community Hospital all the physical therapy equipment are located in one large room. Several patients and their therapists are usually present in the room at the same time. Sometimes family members stay with the patients during the therapy sessions. In this kind of setting, what can be done to maintain confidentiality for individual patients?

References

1. Ronald Munson, "Confidentiality" in *Intervention and Reflection: Basic Issues in Medical Ethics*, 8th ed. ed. Ronald Munson (Belmont, CA: Thomson Wadsworth, 2008).
2. Morton E. Winston, "AIDS, Confidentiality, and The Right to Know," *Public Affairs Quarterly* 2/2 (April 1988): 91–104.
3. Tom L. Beauchamp and LeRoy Walters (eds.), *Contemporary Issues in Bioethics*, 6th ed. (Belmont, CA: Thomson Wadsworth, 2003).
4. Tom L. Beauchamp and James F. Childress, *Principles of Biomedical Ethics*, 5th ed. (New York, NY: Oxford, 2001).
5. California Supreme Court, *Tarasoff v. Regents of the University of California*, 131 *California Reporter* 14 (July 1, 1976).

6. Jill Callahan Dennis, *Privacy and Confidentiality of Health Information* (San Francisco, CA: Jossey-Bass, 2000).

7. Mark Siegler, "Confidentiality in Medicine—A Decrepit Concept," *New England Journal of Medicine* 307/24 (December 9, 1982): 518–21.

8. Ida Critelli Schick, "Protecting Patients' Privacy," *Health Progress* (May–June 1998): 26–31.

9. Maureen Weaver, Jeanette C. Schreiber, Michelle Wilcox DeBarge, Catherine P. Baatz, Wiggin, and Dana, LLP, *The HIPAA Handbook for Implementing the Federal Privacy Rule in the Long-Term Care Setting* (Washington, DC: American Association of Homes and Services for the Aging, 2001).

10. Cynthia Newby, *HIPAA for Allied Health Careers* (New York, NY: McGraw-Hill Higher Education, 2009).

11. University Alliance, University of South Florida Morsoni College of Medicine. "*HITECH Act Summary* http://www.usfhealthonline.com/resources/key-concepts/hitech-act-summary/#.VuDCMOZY4-A Accessed March 2016.

Chapter 13

Workplace Ethics

Many ethical dilemmas in health care are faced by patients and their families. Should a husband and father be taken off a ventilator and allowed to die? When should a "do not resuscitate order" be in place for an elderly patient with Alzheimer's disease? Is abortion permissible when the fetus has a serious genetic defect? Is it ethically permissible to use in vitro fertilization to overcome problems with infertility even though a number of embryos will be lost?

This chapter will have a different focus. It will examine the ethical responsibilities of health care workers themselves and the ethical dilemmas they may face *as employees* of a health care facility.

In this chapter you will learn about:

- The duty of a health care worker to provide care when risk is involved to himself or herself;
- An ethical principle for allocating time and services among patients;
- The ethics of health care workers "using their own judgment" in going against treatment orders for patients they are caring for;

■   A health care worker's ethical responsibilities when a coworker is not doing his or her job.

Case Study

The administration of Memorial Medical Center decides to be proactive in putting a policy into place to deal with epidemics. An ad hoc committee is established to draft a policy. Julia Dunn, a respiratory therapist, is appointed to the committee to represent allied health professionals.

The committee's task is to draft a policy that addresses issues such as working with public health and governmental officials, internal and external communications, education and training for staff, triage, allocation of vaccines and ventilators, and limiting access to the facility (1). When it comes to the human resource issues that must be addressed, Julia feels ambivalent and a bit scared. She is pregnant. In the case of a widespread outbreak of a serious infectious disease, she knows that, as a respiratory therapist, she has special skills that could be much needed and not be provided by other staff. At the same time, she wonders if she would be willing to come to work and risk being infected with a possibly fatal disease, especially while carrying a child.

■   ■   ■

The Duty to Care for Patients

In 1969, the U.S. Surgeon General William Stewart announced to Congress that "it is time to close the book on infectious diseases" (2). Subsequent events proved him to be very wrong in his judgment, most notably, the advent of human immunodeficiency virus (HIV)/acquired immunodeficiency syndrome (AIDS), severe acute respiratory syndrome virus (SARS), and Ebola. Outbreaks of infectious diseases can pose threats to health care workers themselves.

In August 2003, the World Health Organization announced that "20 percent of all persons known to have been infected with SARS were health care workers" (3). Of the 41 people who died of SARS in Canada, three were health care professionals as were 6 of the 180 persons who died of SARS in Taiwan (3). Indeed, "Dr. Carolo Urbani of Medecins Sans Frontieres, who with others initially identified SARS as a new infectious disease in Hanoi, voluntarily quarantined himself and eventually died of SARS, leaving a widow and three children" (3). On the other hand, there were instances during the 2003 SARS outbreak in which some health care professionals "baulked at providing care to those infected with the unknown virus" (4). Sometimes "staffing became an issue in SARS wards and assessment centers; indeed, failure to report for duty during the outbreak resulted in the permanent dismissal of some hospital staff" (4). In sum, the SARS outbreak raised the question of the extent of a health care professional's duty to treat the victims of an outbreak of infectious disease, even at some substantial risk to the caregiver's own health and life (3).

More recently, there has been an outbreak of Ebola in Africa. In 2014, the World Health Organization reported that at least 416 health care workers had contracted Ebola, and that at least 233 had died (5). In the United States, a nurse working at a hospital in Dallas, Texas, contracted Ebola while caring for a Liberian national with the disease (5). A CNN news report on this story raised the question, "What does it feel like to know you're going to treat a patient with a disease that kills 90% of its victims?" (5).

The duty of health care professionals to provide care during an epidemic of an infectious disease is grounded ethically in several considerations.

- The principle of beneficence "recognizes and defines the special moral obligation on the part of HCPs [health care professionals] to further the welfare of patients and to advance patients' well-being" (4) (see Chapter 1).
- The ability and expertise of health care professionals to provide care are greater than that of the general public, thus increasing their obligation to provide care (4).
- By freely choosing a profession devoted to care of the ill, health care professionals have consented to assume a greater than average risk (4).
- In publicly funded health care systems, "there is a strong claim for a social contract between the HCP [health care professional] and society" (4). Specifically, "It is a reasonable and legitimate expectation by the public that HCPs will respond in an infectious disease emergency" (4).

On the other hand, there is recognition that an individual who is a health care professional likely functions in various roles—as spouse, parent, caregiver for relatives—and that these additional roles also carry ethical obligations (4, 6). For example, health care workers have a duty to care for their own children during an epidemic by protecting them (and hence themselves) from infection (6). Or, consider the following case of a health care professional. . .

> who is caring for an elderly parent in her home. Told to come to work in the face of a pandemic that could result in her being quarantined within the hospital for an indefinite period of time, and where her life

would be put at risk, is she a bad person if she weighs her professional obligations against her duties to care for those who depend upon her at home?

According to McCullough's analysis, a health provider who could simply abandon her mother at home in the name of adhering to an abstract professional duty might not be the sort of human being we would wish to care for us . . . (3)

Moreover, health care professionals surely have "obligations to themselves and to their own health (particularly those with special vulnerabilities, such as a comorbid condition)" (4).

In sum, health care professionals may have personal obligations to others and to themselves, which conflict with their professional duty to provide care for patients during an outbreak of an infectious disease. This suggests that, while there is in general a duty on the part of health care workers to provide care to patients, this duty is limited and may have legitimate exceptions (6). One strategy may be to allow certain cases in which a health care professional is considered exempt from coming to work during an epidemic of an infectious disease, perhaps being placed on furlough (1). Short of this solution, policies may be put into place to reassign health care workers with special needs (e.g., female health care workers who are pregnant) to low-risk duties, such as caring for patients who do not have the infectious disease or assuming administrative duties that do not involve patient care (1). Or again, creative solutions might be developed for meeting both professional and personal duties. For example, an assistance program might be put into place to provide care at home for relatives of health care workers, making it more likely for them to come to work (3). The discussion of how to resolve this conflict between professional and personal duties is ongoing (3, 6)

Case Study

David Stock is a physical therapist who comes weekly to Stoneridge Manor to provide physical therapy services for its residents. Stoneridge is a multi-level facility for retired persons consisting of independent living apartments, assisted living units, and a nursing home unit.

David is currently providing physical therapy for three residents, Wanda Taylor, Fred Sullivan, and Mark Kohl. Before he visits these residents, he stops by the office of the director of nursing (DON) to get an update on their conditions.

Wanda is residing in the independent living apartments. The DON tells David that Wanda's daughter is making a trip today from another state to see her mother and is bringing her children with her. They plan to take Wanda out to lunch. Because of the long driving distance, they are not sure at exactly what time they will arrive that morning.

Fred is in the nursing home unit. The DON tells David that Fred has been experiencing considerable discomfort in his left leg for several days to the point of needing additional pain medication. The DON hopes that physical therapy will make him more comfortable.

Mark resides in the assisted living unit. Mark is the kind of person who has gone by a schedule all his life. He gets very upset when things get "off schedule," and this emotional stress aggravates his problem with high blood pressure. Mark is normally the first resident David treats, promptly at 11:00 a.m.

While David is having this conversation with the DON, the DON receives a call that a resident, Amanda Miller, has choked on a piece of hard candy she wasn't supposed to have in the first place and that she has stopped breathing. Resuscitation is needed immediately. David has been trained in cardiopulmonary resuscitation (CPR).

How should David handle this situation in terms of his caregiving responsibilities?

■ ■ ■

Allocating Staff Time and Services Among Patients

The time and services of health care workers are resources that must sometimes be allocated. Especially when there is a staffing shortage, health care workers may be faced with decisions about which patient should receive care first. Ethically, these allocation decisions involve *distributive justice*, the principle concerned with fairness in the distribution of benefits, burdens, and resources (see Chapter 1).

Philosophers have tried to spell out more concretely how benefits and resources are distributed fairly. One interpretation given to distributive justice is the *principle of equality*, according to which "everyone is to be treated the same in all respects" (7). More simply stated, this interpretation of distributive justice maintains that "everyone is entitled to the same size slice of the pie" (7). Another interpretation of distributive justice is the *principle of contribution*, according to which "everyone should get back that proportion of social goods that is the result of his or her productive labor" (7). If one person works twice as hard or long as a second, the first person should be entitled to twice as large a share in the benefits (7). The interpretation of distributive justice that is most likely relevant to the situation of health care workers is the *principle of need*:

> The principle of need is an extension of the egalitarian principle of equal distribution. If goods are parceled out according to individual need, those who have greater needs will receive a greater share. However, the outcome will be one of equality. Since the basic needs of everyone will be met, everyone will end up at the same level. The treatment of individuals will be equal, in this respect, even though the proportion of goods they receive will not be. (7)

Thus, if two (or more) patients need attention, a health care worker should prioritize his or her services and time according to which patient has the greater (greatest) need.

Let us apply the principle of need to the decisions David Stock has to make. First, David has to decide between giving physical therapy to Wanda, Fred, and Mark (the reason he came to Stoneridge Manor) and administering CPR to Amanda, the resident who choked on a piece of candy. Amanda is in a life-threatening situation, whereas Wanda, Fred, and Mark are not. Clearly, the resident who choked and needs resuscitation has the greatest need. If no one else who is adequately trained in CPR is immediately available, David should respond to Amanda first.

The problem is that many decisions about allocating time and services are not this clear. Suppose that the DON can attend to Amanda, allowing David to proceed with the physical therapy services for which he came to Stoneridge Manor. Mark is probably already upset that David is late to administer his physical therapy, and this is not good for his blood pressure. While Mark is experiencing emotional distress, Fred has been experiencing serious physical discomfort. Physical therapy may well help relieve the discomfort he has been experiencing for several days. And on the other hand, if David does not attend to Wanda right away, her daughter may come to take her to lunch before David can get to her. If Wanda misses her physical therapy entirely, this is likely to result in physical discomfort for her later in the week. Which of these residents should David attend to first? Whose need is the greatest?

If Fred is presently experiencing serious discomfort, we would likely judge his need to be the greatest. On the other hand, if his discomfort is being adequately managed through pain medication, he could probably wait a bit to have his physical therapy administered.

Case Study

Julie Ames works as a dietitian at Spring Valley Home. Part of her job is making sure that dietary restrictions for particular residents are observed. Because of heart problems, George Mason's doctor has put him on a low-fat, low-sodium diet. George usually cooperates without too much complaint, but he loves sweet corn and "just can't eat it without some salt." Spring Valley always has a picnic for residents on the Fourth of July, and this year a local farmer—in fact, a friend of George—has donated a truckload of sweet corn to the home for the picnic. Julie knows that George will feel left out and hurt if he isn't served sweet corn, especially since it comes from a personal friend. She also knows that if George is served the sweet corn plain, he will raise a fuss with the staff about getting some salt. A conflict between George and the staff during the picnic will ruin the day for both him and the staff. Julie decides to tell a dietary aide to put two packets of salt onto George's tray. After all, this one breach of his diet shouldn't harm him.

■ ■ ■

We might then consider the needs of Wanda to be the most urgent. After all, it may be a case of Wanda receiving therapy now or forgoing it entirely for that week. Mark will eventually receive his therapy, the only question is when.

At the same, Mark's emotional distress cannot be totally discounted. Indeed, this may aggravate his high blood pressure. Mark, too, has a real need. In this case, a solution might be found to meet the needs of both Wanda and Mark. Before seeing Wanda, perhaps David could stop into Mark's room to calm him down by explaining the needs of other residents that require his attention, and reassuring him that he will be back to administer his therapy as soon as he is able.

Staff Who "Use Their Own Judgment"

In this case, a staff member of a health care facility takes it upon herself to do something for a resident that directly goes against the orders of a physician. The staff member makes the judgment that the resident's health will not be harmed by going against the physician's orders. Ethically, is it permissible for staff to act in this way?

Some would approach this case not by looking at the behavior of staff, but rather, by focusing on residents and their autonomy. Allowing a person to direct the course of his or her own life is a value much emphasized in contemporary health care ethics. Thus, some would argue that the proper course of action is to explain to George the possible consequences for his heart condition of using salt, but to allow him to make the decision whether he wishes to take those risks. Once health care providers have informed George of the risks and are confident that he understands them and is mentally competent to make decisions, then both the physician and the nursing home staff should abide by George's wishes, even if they personally disagree with his choice. If George wants salt for his sweet corn, he should have it! (8).

However, not everyone would place such an exclusive emphasis on patient autonomy. They would point out that health care providers have a duty of *nonmaleficence*, a duty not to take actions that cause or risk harm to patients. In the case of George, autonomy and nonmaleficence may be in conflict (see Chapter 1). In other words, there may be a conflict between what George wants to do in terms of eating and what his doctor believes would further harm his already fragile health.

The question can be raised whether Julie the dietitian violated the ethical duty of nonmaleficence in providing salt for George. She "used her own judgment" in believing that George would not be harmed by her action. But can she really be so sure that she has the professional knowledge to make these assessments on her own?

If staff member Julie questioned the wisdom of an absolute prohibition of salt seasoning for George, it would have been more appropriate for her to raise this question with George's physician or at a care conference for George. Bringing this question out into the open would provide the opportunity to discuss whether occasional indulgences in salt seasoning would in fact be harmful to George's health. After discussion, perhaps George's physician would agree to occasional indulgences.

Case Study

Rhonda Lewis is a registered nurse who has worked for 10 years at Spring Valley Home. She is known as a good worker and as someone who is very conscientious. Rhonda has some concerns about Jerry Miles who comes every week to administer physical therapy to some of the residents of Spring Valley Home. Several times, she has smelled alcohol on Jerry's breath. On one occasion she walked into George Mason's room and found

Jerry helping him with exercises for his legs. The problem is that George did not need these exercises. Jerry was supposed to give them to the man in the room next to George's. George wasn't at all hurt by this mistake, but Rhonda wonders how often this kind of mistake is occurring. Another resident, Henry Thompson, has complained to her that Jerry has skipped him on several occasions. And when Henry does not get his exercises, he gets stiff and experiences some difficulty in walking. Rhonda wonders what she should do. She has always believed that coworkers should not "rat" on each other. And she knows how difficult it is to get outside health care workers to provide services at a nursing home, especially on a weekly basis. What will the residents of Spring Valley Home do if they lose Jerry?

■ ■ ■

Problems With the Job Performance of Coworkers

In this case, Rhonda is concerned about the job performance of a coworker, Jerry, who comes to Spring Valley Home to administer physical therapy to some of the residents. The ethical duty of beneficence tells Rhonda that she must act to prevent harm from coming to the residents of Spring Valley Home (see Chapter 1). She has caught one mistake Jerry made on the job, giving exercises to the wrong resident. In this case, the mistake did not cause the resident any harm. But if this sort of mistake occurs again, it is possible that a resident could suffer from the unneeded exercises. Also, Jerry has caused discomfort to another resident on several occasions by forgetting about his therapy altogether. In addition, Rhonda worries about the fact that she has smelled alcohol on Jerry's breath several times. She knows that alcohol can impair performance and cause someone to make mistakes. The situation with Jerry presents the potential for harm. Therefore, the duty of beneficence entails that Rhonda cannot just let this situation slip by, but is morally obligated to take action.

Rhonda has strong feelings that coworkers should not "rat" on each other. Perhaps, then, the first step is for Rhonda to confront Jerry himself with her concerns about his job performance. Is it the case that Jerry has made mistakes and been forgetful because of a stressful situation within his own family that is only temporary? Or are his mistakes and forgetfulness due to a more enduring problem? What is the cause of Jerry's apparent alcohol abuse? On his own, will Jerry decide to get appropriate professional help if needed?

In her job, Rhonda's first obligation is to the residents of Spring Valley Home and to promoting their welfare and protecting them from harm. If Rhonda's conversation with Jerry does not result in a change of job performance, or if Rhonda does not feel comfortable about having such a conversation with Jerry, then she has an obligation to report this situation to her supervisor. Although she may not want to "rat" on Jerry, her obligation to prevent harm to residents takes precedence over her feelings.

CHAPTER SUMMARY

Key Terms and Concepts

principle of patient autonomy: self-determination; an individual's right to hold views, make choices, and take actions based on personal values and beliefs.

principle of beneficence: the ethical duty to act in ways that help people and promote their welfare; this includes preventing evil and harm, removing evil and harm, and doing or promoting good.

principle of nonmaleficence: the ethical duty to act in ways that do not cause harm to people.

principle of distributive justice: fairness in the distribution of benefits, burdens, and resources.

principle of need: an interpretation of distributive justice giving priority in the distribution of resources to those with the greatest need.

Key Points

- In general, health care workers have a professional duty to provide care for patients, even in cases (such as an outbreak of an infectious disease) posing risk to their own health and life. However, this duty may be limited by personal obligations of the health care workers.
- Because of staffing shortages, health care workers may have to make decisions about which patients to help and which ones must have care postponed, at least temporarily. Ethically, a guiding principle is the *principle of need*, directing health care workers to prioritize their time and services according to which patient has the greater (greatest) need.
- Health care workers have a duty of nonmaleficence, that is, a duty to act in ways that do not cause harm or pose a risk of harm to patients. Health care workers should be cautious about "using their own judgment" in ways that go against the course of treatment prescribed for a patient. If a health care worker believes that the prescribed course of treatment is not in the

patient's best interests, he or she should raise this issue with a supervisor, with the patient's physician, or at a care conference.

■ When a health care worker observes job performance problems with coworkers (for example, treatment mistakes, failure to do the job at all, impairment due to substance abuse) which may bring harm to patients, the duty of beneficence requires him or her to take preventive action. This may mean alerting supervisors to the job performance problem.

FOR FURTHER DISCUSSION

1. In this chapter we have discussed the extreme case of a health care worker's obligation to come to work in the event of an epidemic of an infectious disease. But consider the following scenario:

> Brigid O'Connor is the director of radiologic services at St. Luke's Hospital. Among her duties, she is responsible for seeing that there is adequate staffing. On several occasions, she has called in Sally Furtweiler, one of the technologists in the department. Sally frequently telephones at the last minute to say that she cannot come to work that day. On one occasion, she said she had car trouble. On another occasion, she had an emergency dental appointment. On more than one occasion, she has said she cannot come to work because of a sick child or because of bad weather. Then there was the time Sally didn't come in because her sister came to visit from California. Brigid is tempted to fire Sally for excessive absenteeism, but she does do so because of the staffing shortage health care facilities in that geographical area are experiencing. Brigid reasons that having Sally work part of the time is better than nothing!
>
> However, Sally's absence from work unexpectedly and frequently presents a staffing problem. Roy Taylor works with Sally on the same shift, and Roy has complained to Brigid several times about not being able to take care of all the patients properly when Sally is absent.
>
> On one occasion, when Roy was the only radiographer on duty, he took an X-ray that showed the patient to have an enlarged heart. When this was reported to the patient, she became very distressed. This patient has problems with high blood pressure, and her anxiety over the results of the x-ray only aggravated her problem. Further diagnostic testing showed that the x-ray picture had been faulty, probably because Roy was in such a hurry to take it.

On that same occasion, the fact that "one person had to do the work of two" caused a delay in Roy responding to a request for x-rays in the emergency room (ER). This, in turn, caused a delay in treating the patient.

We would all agree that there are emergency situations that make absence from work necessary and justified. However, it seems that Sally Furtweiler is not taking her duty to come to work seriously enough.

In what circumstances do you think it is legitimate for a health care worker to decide not to come to work? Is bad weather a legitimate reason? Caring for a sick child? Personal illness? An emergency dental appointment?

Hint: Try using the utilitarian ethical theory in working through these questions, looking at the consequences for everyone who will be affected by the course of action (see Chapter 1).

2. Pam Hays is a respiratory therapist at Westridge Hospital. Because of an outbreak of flu, she is the only respiratory therapist currently on duty. Her two coworkers have called in sick.

   John Wright has been hospitalized for emphysema, but is scheduled to be released this morning. Pam is scheduled to give him therapy at 9:00 a.m. before he leaves for home.

   When Pam is on her way to see John, she is paged to go to the ER. Instinctively she does this, where she is asked to set up a ventilator for a patient who has just been brought to the ER. While she is doing this, a nurse tells her that a mother has just come to the ER with a child who has cystic fibrosis. The mother is concerned that the therapy she did at home that morning with her son did not adequately clear the mucus from his lungs. She has taken time off from work to bring her son to the ER but needs to return to work as soon as possible.

   Pam, a mother herself, sympathizes with this woman's concerns about her son and appreciates the time constraints she is under with respect to her job. At the same time, Pam knows that she has the scheduled appointment with Mr. Wright, and that his wife is coming to take him home shortly. Pam is faced with a dilemma: Should she next attend to the boy with cystic fibrosis or to Mr. Wright?

   In your judgment, whom should Pam see next? What are the reasons behind your judgment?

3. Ted Collins is on the dietary staff at Spring Valley Home. He smokes heavily. He does not smoke in the facility itself, but whenever he gets a break from his work in the kitchen, he goes outside and lights up. A coworker, Jill Pierce, is upset with Ted for doing this. She tells him that residents who are walking or sitting outdoors can see him smoke and that this tempts residents who are restricted from smoking for health reasons. Jill tells her supervisor that Ted should be made to give up smoking entirely while at work.

   - *Is this situation different from the case of Jerry Miles, who showed up at Spring Valley Home to administer physical therapy with alcohol on his breath?*
   - *Jill's complaints to her supervisor would be legitimate and would fall under the duty of beneficence if Ted's behavior at work poses a threat of harm to the residents. Can a case be made that Ted is harming residents by his smoking?*

4. Suppose that you are asked to serve on an ad hoc committee to develop the specific criteria for the annual staff evaluation process. What specific standards would you suggest for the areas of absence from work, following treatment directives for patients and handling job performance problems with coworkers? And why would you suggest these particular standards?

References

1. Centers for Disease Control and Prevention, "*HHS Pandemic Influenza Plan Supplement 3 Healthcare Planning.*" http://www.col.ops-oms.org/servicios/influenza/reunion/docs/CDC_planeacion_hospitalaria.pdf. Accessed February 2016.
2. Daniel K. Sokol, "*Doctors' first duty: Professional or personal?*" *International Herald Tribune* (October 21, 2005). http://medicalethicist.net. Accessed June 2016.
3. Howard Brody and Eric N. Avery, "Medicine's Duty to Treat Pandemic Illness Solidarity and Vulnerability," *Hastings Center Report* 39/1 (January–February 2009): 40–48.
4. Carly Ruderman, C. Shawn Tracy, Cecile M. Bensimon, Mark Bernstein, Laura Hawryluck, Randi Zlotnik Shaul, and Ross EG Upshur, "On Pandemics and the Duty to Care: Whose Duty? Whose Care?" *BMC Medical Ethics* 7/5 (2006). http://www.biomedcentral.com/1472-6939/7/5. Accessed February 2016.
5. Ashley Fantz, "For Ebola Caregivers, Enormous Fear, Risk and Bravery." CNN October 12, 2014. http://www.cnn.com/2014/10/12/health/ebola-health-care-workers. Accessed February 2016.

6. Daniel K. Sokol, "Virulent Epidemics and Scope of Healthcare Workers' Duty of Care," *Emerging Infectious Diseases* 12/8 (August 2006). http://wwwnc.cdc.gov /eid/article/12/8/06-0360_article. Accessed February 2016.

7. Ronald Munson, "Principles of Distributive Justice" in *Intervention and Reflection: Basic Issues in Medical Ethics*, 8th ed. ed. Ronald Munson (Belmont, CA: Thomson Wadsworth, 2008).

8. "Beyond the Call of Duty: A Nurse's Aide Uses Her Judgment" in *Everyday Ethics: Resolving Dilemmas in Nursing Home Life*, eds. Rosalie Kane and Arthur L. Caplan (New York, NY: Springer, 1990).

Chapter 14

Ethical and Religious Objections to Health Care Practices

Health care treatments and interventions can be ethically and religiously controversial. The abortion debate in the United States is a prime example of this. Some people favor assisted suicide, whereas others are opposed to it on ethical and religious grounds. Some have objections in conscience to such practices as in vitro fertilization and the freezing of embryos. While most people in American society take blood transfusions for granted, Jehovah's Witnesses refuse them on religious grounds.

Patients will bring their ethical and religious values with them when seeking health care services. Similarly, health care workers also have personal beliefs about what is right and wrong to do.

In this chapter you will learn about:

- The right of an adult patient to refuse a medical treatment on ethical or religious grounds;

■ The scope of parental authority to refuse a medical treatment for a child because of ethical or religious objections to it;

■ The right of a health care worker to be excused from participating in a treatment or course of action to which he or she has ethical or religious objections.

Case Study

Rebecca Stanton, 43, is an outpatient at the cancer treatment center of St. Margaret's Medical Center. She is undergoing radiation treatments for a small cancerous tumor in her stomach. The prospects for the cancer going into remission look good. Extensive examination also indicates a preleukemic blood condition, but Rebecca's physician is confident that this can be successfully treated with monthly blood transfusions.

When Rebecca is approached about beginning the blood transfusions, she unqualifiedly refuses. She states that she is a Jehovah's Witness and that her religion does not permit blood transfusions. She says that she will put her faith in God. "If God wants me to continue to live," she states, "I will recover without the blood transfusions."

St. Margaret's is a Catholic-sponsored facility, a religious tradition that accepts the practice of blood transfusions. The oncology staff at St. Margaret's cannot understand how there can be *religious* reasons for refusing a blood transfusion that clearly will be beneficial to someone's health.

Rebecca has taken a special liking to one radiation therapist, Barbara Baxter. Several members of the oncology staff ask Barbara to talk to Rebecca about the transfusions. Barbara poses to Rebecca a situation in which she thinks it will be impossible for Rebecca to condemn transfusions. "Think back to the time when your son was just five years old," Barbara tells Rebecca, "and was injured in an automobile accident. Suppose that your son had been so severely injured that he would die unless he had a blood transfusion. As a mother, wouldn't you have wanted the transfusion to save your son's life?" To Barbara's surprise, Rebecca calmly replies that she could have accepted her son's death as God's will.

At this point, Barbara Baxter and several other staff members ask to meet with the hospital's ethics committee to help them deal with this baffling situation.

■ ■ ■

Objections to Health Care Practices by Patients and Families

Perhaps the classic case of a religious objection to a medical practice is the refusal of blood transfusions by Jehovah's Witnesses. This refusal is based on Old Testament texts, such as Genesis 9:4, Leviticus 3:17 and 7:26, and Acts 15:28–29, which forbid "partaking of any blood" (1, 2).

A famous court case involving the refusal of blood transfusions by a Jehovah's Witness is *In re Brooks Estate* from the state of Illinois. In May 1964, Bernice Brooks was in McNeal General Hospital in Chicago suffering from a peptic ulcer. She was attended by Dr. Gilbert Demange and had informed him repeatedly during a 2-year period prior to her hospitalization that her religious beliefs prevented her from receiving blood transfusions. In fact, Mrs. Brooks and her husband signed a document releasing Dr. Demange and the hospital from all civil liability that might result from a failure to administer blood transfusions to Mrs. Brooks. Despite this, Dr. Demange, together with several assistant State's attorneys and the attorney for the public guardian of Cook County, Illinois, appeared before the probate division of the circuit court with a petition by the public guardian requesting appointment of the guardian as a conservator of Bernice Brooks. Further, the petition requested an order authorizing the conservator to consent to the administration of blood to Mrs. Brooks. The court appointed the conservator and a blood transfusion was administered to Mrs. Brooks (3).

This situation involved a conflict between what the patient wanted (namely, no blood transfusions) and what the physician felt obligated to do for the welfare of the patient. Ethically speaking, this situation involved a conflict between *patient autonomy* and the health care professional's duty of *beneficence* (see Chapter 1).

The Illinois court made the following judgment in this case:

> . . . It seems to be clearly established that the First Amendment of the United States Constitution, as extended to the individual States by the Fourteenth Amendment to that Constitution, protects the absolute right of every individual to freedom in his religious belief and the exercise thereof, subject only to the qualification that the exercise thereof may be properly limited by governmental action where such exercise endangers, clearly and presently, the public health, welfare or morals.
>
> . . . No overt or affirmative act of appellants offers any clear and present danger to society—we have only a governmental agency compelling conduct offensive to appellant's religious principles. Even though we may consider appellant's beliefs unwise, foolish or ridiculous, in the absence of an overriding danger to society we may not permit

interference therewith in the form of a conservatorship established in the waning hours of her life for the sole purpose of compelling her to accept medical treatment forbidden by her religious principles and previously refused by her with full knowledge of the probable consequences. In the final analysis, what has happened here involves a judicial attempt to decide what course of action is best for a particular individual, notwithstanding that individual's contrary views based upon religious convictions. Such action cannot be constitutionally countenanced. (3)

The Illinois court took the position that an individual's religious freedom must be respected and can only be limited when the person's behavior threatens harm to society. Thus, Mrs. Brooks had the right to refuse blood transfusions on religious grounds, and it was wrong for a conservator to have been appointed to force blood transfusions on her.

In the case of Mrs. Brooks, the Illinois court came down on the side of patient autonomy. Several arguments might be put forward to support giving priority to individual autonomy in this case (see Chapter 1).

First, patients other than Jehovah's Witnesses can and do make the choice not to follow their physician's recommendations. In one study, "19% of patients at teaching hospitals refused at least one treatment or procedure, even though 15% of such refusals were potentially life endangering" (4). Generalizing this point, refusing a medical procedure on religious grounds can be seen as one instance of the phenomenon of patient choice regarding medical treatments.

Moreover, there are other cases in which therapies have to be altered to accommodate special circumstances, such as hypertension, severe allergy to antibiotics, or the unavailability of certain costly equipment (4). Analogously, when a patient objects to a particular medical treatment on religious grounds, health care providers "are being asked to manage the medical or surgical problem in harmony with the patient's choice and conscience" (4).

Finally, health care providers should keep in mind the psychological damage that may be inflicted on a patient by forcing her to undergo a medical treatment against her conscience:

> If a court forced an abhorrent treatment on you, how might this affect your conscience and the vital element of your will to live? Dr. Konrad Drebinger wrote: "It would certainly be a misguided form of medical ambition that would lead one to force a patient to accept a given therapy, overruling his conscience, so as to treat him physically but dealing his psyche a mortal blow." (2)

In other words, the focus should be on treating "the whole person" (5).

The case study of Rebecca Stanton hypothesizes a scenario in which her son would need a blood transfusion after being seriously injured in an auto accident. This scenario differs in one important respect from the case of Mrs. Brooks. Rebecca's son is only 5 years old, and the decision to forgo a blood transfusion would be made by his parents. While it is recognized that a mentally competent adult patient who has been adequately informed of the potential advantages and risks of a proposed treatment does have the right to refuse it, even when the best medical opinion deems it essential to save the patient's life (6, 7), it is another issue whether parents can legitimately make this decision for a child who is incapable of deciding for himself (8).

While there is a presumption in favor of parental decision-making authority for their children, the parental authority is not absolute. Legally, children fall under the *parens patriae* power of the state as persons unable to protect themselves (9). In the exercise of this power, the state may step in before parental decisions "become operative to ensure that the choices made are not so detrimental to a child's interests as to amount to neglect and abuse" (9). Parents are considered to be "under obligation to provide minor children with the necessities of life, which includes medical care deemed necessary to prevent children's deaths" (10). And, "if any or all of this is not performed, the principles of law override professed religious convictions of the parents" (10). As stated by the Superior Court of the State of Illinois:

> Parents may be free to become martyrs themselves. It does not follow, however, that they are free in identical circumstances to make martyrs of their children before they have reached an age of full and legal discretion, when they can make that choice for themselves. Laws, while they cannot interfere with religious belief and opinion, may be constitutionally appropriate for interfering with religious practices. (11)

If a child of Jehovah's Witnesses requires a blood transfusion, a court could intervene and appoint a legal guardian other than the child's parents who would authorize the transfusion (11). Indeed, one court "took the view that a judicially ordered blood transfusion could properly be administered to a pregnant patient, when such was necessary to save her life, even though she and her husband had refused to authorize transfusions because of their religious beliefs, upon the grounds that it would be justified in the interest of protecting the unborn child . . ." (11).

In sum, St. Margaret's Medical Center would be obliged to treat the cases of Rebecca Stanton and of her son differently. While staff could try to persuade Rebecca to have the needed blood transfusions, they would be required to respect her wishes to decline them if that were her ultimate decision. On the other hand, if Rebecca refused the needed blood transfusions for her son, the staff could pursue legal action, asking for a legal guardian other than his parents to be appointed to make the medical treatment decisions (6).

What has been said about the case of Jehovah's Witnesses and refusal of blood transfusions would apply to other cases of religious objections to health care treatments and interventions. For example, it would apply to those who reject "standard" medical treatment in favor of faith-healing services.

Case Study

Terry Welsh is a new respiratory therapist at St. Margaret's Medical Center. He is very active in a local pro-life group. He has strong feelings that it is morally wrong to withhold or withdraw life-sustaining treatments. This is, he believes, just a way of "getting rid of people who are difficult or whose care is expensive." He is also against advance directives because they allow forgoing life-sustaining treatments. In fact, he has a stack of pamphlets warning against advance directives, and he has been known to pass them out to patients and families at the hospital.

John Springer, who is in the final stages of Alzheimer's disease and also suffers from chronic pulmonary disease, has been transferred from a nursing home to St. Margaret's because he has developed pneumonia. Antibiotic treatment and ventilator support are initiated. Several days passed, but John does not appear to improve.

A durable power of attorney for health care executed by John names his wife, Louise, as his proxy decision maker. After talking with their children, Louise tells John's physician that she wants the antibiotics and ventilator support stopped. Alzheimer's disease is a terminal condition, she says, and John is at the stage where he can no longer enjoy life because he is bedridden and suffering from severe dementia. "John would never want to live like this," she states. She believes it is time that the natural dying process should be allowed to take its course. After all, pneumonia is "the old person's friend." John's physician agrees with her.

Terry Welsh is instructed by John's physician to disconnect the ventilator. However, Terry tells his supervisor that John's family and physician are "killing him" by not administering antibiotics and by withdrawing the ventilator, and that his conscience will not allow him to be a part of this affair. "On moral grounds," he tells his supervisor, "I can no longer be involved in John's case."

■ ■ ■

Objections of Conscience by Health Care Workers

Health care workers may sometimes be asked to perform a procedure or participate in a course of action to which they personally object on ethical or religious
grounds. A common case is the participation of health care workers in abortion
procedures. But this is not the only kind of situation in which objections of conscience can arise. In this case, Terry, a respiratory therapist, firmly believes it is
morally wrong to withhold or withdraw life-sustaining treatments, and refuses to
participate in the care of John Springer, a patient with pneumonia from whom
antibiotics and ventilator support are to be withdrawn by the choice of his
proxy decision maker. In Terry's mind, an action on his part of disconnecting
John's ventilator would be participating in the process of deliberately causing a
patient's death.

It is recognized that health care facilities can legitimately refuse to provide what a patient (or his proxy decision maker) may want. As stated by the
Special Committee on Biomedical Ethics of the American Hospital Association,
"Generally, a hospital may refuse to provide a service to a patient if the procedure is inappropriate to its mission (e.g., therapeutic abortion, artificial insemination)" (12). Similarly, the federal *Patient Self-Determination Act* on advance
directives contains a conscience clause. With respect to complying with the
directives set out by a patient in a living will or durable power of attorney for
health care, no facility is required to act contrary to its own mission and ethical
values. However, a health care facility must have clearly written policies specifying the limits on the procedures it will perform and make this information available to its clients (13).

Similarly, it is recognized that health care workers have a right to refuse to
participate in procedures and courses of action to which they personally have
ethical or religious objections. As stated by the Special Committee on Biomedical
Ethics of the American Hospital Association:

> If a patient chooses a course of treatment that is not acceptable to the
> attending physician or other health care professionals, those individu-
> als may withdraw from the case, as long as doing so does not amount
> to legal abandonment. If a suitably qualified alternative physician or
> health care professional willing to comply with the patient's preference
> is available, transfer to the care of that individual should be offered to
> the patient. (12)

Thus, if Terry believes it is ethically wrong to forgo life-sustaining treatments
(in this case, antibiotics and ventilator support for pneumonia), he should be

allowed to withdraw from being involved in the care of John Springer, with another respiratory therapist taking his place. However, there are several provisos for this concession to Terry.

First, Terry has an obligation to make known his refusal of treatment "in advance and in time for other appropriate arrangements to be made" for the care of the patient (14). Terry knows that instances of withholding or withdrawing life-sustaining treatments are likely to occur in a hospital setting. He has an obligation to let his supervisor know about his ethical stance *before* he is faced with the case of John Springer. After all, the hospital will have to make arrangements for another respiratory therapist to take Terry's place in caring for John. If Terry suddenly announces his ethical objections to participating in withdrawing the ventilator, the hospital may not be able to locate a substitute respiratory therapist and John's dying process may be prolonged and his wife may be distressed.

Second, Terry must make sure that his refusal to participate in withdrawing the ventilator is based on accurate and complete information (14, 15). Terry believes that withholding or withdrawing life-sustaining treatments is just a way of "getting rid of people who are difficult or whose care is expensive." But does he really understand what people's motivation can be for forgoing life-sustaining treatments? The motivation of John's wife seems to be that she does not want to prolong her husband's suffering and that John himself would not want to live completely bedridden and with severe dementia. Does Terry recognize the emotional strain John's wife may be experiencing in "letting go" of her husband? Does Terry understand that there is a difference between forgoing life-sustaining treatments and involuntary euthanasia (which may be an attempt to "get rid of people")? Is he familiar with what ethicists and religious denominations are saying about the permissibility of forgoing life-sustaining treatments? In sum, before Terry can legitimately voice an objection of conscience to participating in withdrawing the ventilator, he has an obligation to become factually and ethically informed about withholding and withdrawing life-sustaining treatments.

Suppose that Terry persists in his belief that it is ethically wrong to withhold or withdraw life-sustaining treatments. He may have to consider changing his place of employment. It is undoubtedly a policy of St. Margaret's Medical Center to allow patients to forgo life-sustaining treatments. If it becomes a frequent occurrence that a substitute worker has to be found for Terry because of his objections of conscience and if this proves difficult for Terry's supervisor to do, then Terry's job performance may be called into question. In this case, it may be best for Terry to seek employment at a facility holding ethical views more similar to his own. It is nothing new to say that there may be a price to pay for adhering to one's ethical principles.

CHAPTER SUMMARY

Key Terms and Concepts

principle of autonomy: self-determination; an individual's right to hold views, make choices, and take actions based on personal values and beliefs.

principle of beneficence: the ethical duty to act in ways that help people and promote their welfare; this includes preventing evil and harm, removing evil and harm, and doing or promoting good.

Key Points

- An adult patient who is mentally competent and who has been adequately informed of the potential advantages and risks of a medical treatment does have the right to refuse it. The grounds for refusal may be ethical or religious, even if these beliefs are not accepted by other people.
- Parents cannot make the same kinds of decisions about refusing medical treatment for their children that they can make for themselves. Under the *parens patriae* power of the state, types of medical treatment can be legally mandated for children even though the parents find them ethically or religiously objectionable.
- A health care facility can legitimately refuse to provide to a patient a service that goes against the facility's mission and ethical values.
- Health care workers have a right to refuse to participate in procedures and courses of action that go against their ethical principles and religious beliefs. However, this refusal should be made known in advance and in time for other arrangements to be made for patient care.
- Objections of conscience are responsibly made by health care workers only if they are based on accurate and complete information about the facts of the case and about relevant ethical principles.
- For the sake of satisfactory job performance, a health care worker who has ethical or religious objections to a procedure or course of action allowed by the facility's policies may be faced with the decision of seeking employment at another facility.

FOR FURTHER DISCUSSION

1. Are there any religious groups (e.g., Christian Scientists) in your geographical area whose beliefs may affect their acceptance of "standard" health care practices, procedures, and technologies? How much do you know about the beliefs of such groups?

2. Are there any procedures or courses of action in caring for patients that you yourself find ethically objectionable? Religiously objectionable? If so, what are the grounds on which you find them objectionable? Do you think that your ethical or religious views may cause you to run into any problems in your job or role in health care? Can you think of a means to accommodate your objections of conscience while still doing your job or fulfilling your role satisfactorily?

3. Courts have the power to arrange for medical treatments for children even though their parents find them ethically or religiously objectionable. Do you think that courts ought to have this power or that parental decision-making authority on behalf of their children should be absolute? How would you feel if legal measures were taken to initiate a medical treatment on one of your children against your wishes?

References

1. Orville N. Griese, *Catholic Identity in Health Care: Principles and Practice* (Braintree, MA: Pope John Center, 1987).

2. Jehovah's Witnesses Official Web Site, "*You Have the Right to Choose.*" http://www.jw.org/en/publications/books/blood/you-have-the-right-to-choose. Accessed February 2016.

3. Emory C. Underwood, "From *In re Brooks Estate*" in *Experimentation With Human Beings*, ed. J. Katz (New York: Russell Sage Foundation, 1972).

4. Dixon J. Lowell, "Blood: Whose Choice and Whose Conscience?" *New York State Journal of Medicine* 88 (1988): 463–64.

5. J.L. Dixon and M.G. Smalley "Jehovah's Witnesses: The Surgical/Ethical Challenge," *Journal of the American Medical Association* 246/21 (November 27, 1981): 2471–72.

6. Laurance T. Wren, "Status of the Law on Medical and Religious Conflicts in Blood Transfusions," *Arizona Medicine* 24 (October 1967): 970–73.

7. David H. Wilson, "Patients' Wishes Must Be Accepted," *British Medical Journal* 308 (28 May 1994): 1424.

8. Baruch Brody, Commentary on "Faith Healing for Childhood Leukemia" in *Cases in Bioethics: Selections from the Hastings Center Report,* 3rd ed. ed. Bette-Jane Crigger (New York: St. Martin's Press, 1998).

9. President's Commission for the Study of Ethical Problems in Medicine and Biomedical and Behavioral Research, *Deciding to Forego Life-Sustaining Treatment* (March 1983; reprint New York: Concern for Dying).

10. J.W. Holloway, Jr., "Blood Transfusions—Jehovah's Witnesses," *Journal of the American Medical Association* 163 (1957): 660, quoted in 11 below.

11. George Thomas, Robert W. Edmark, and Thomas Jones, "Issues Involved With Surgery of Jehovah's Witnesses," *The American Surgeon* 34/7 (July 1968): 542–43.

12. Special Committee on Biomedical Ethics, *Values in Conflict Resolving Ethical Issues in Hospital Care* (Chicago, IL: American Hospital Association, 1985).

13. Catholic Health Association of the United States, *The Patient Self-Determination Act* (St. Louis, MO: Catholic Health Association of the United States, 1991).

14. Ellen W. Bernal and Patricia S. Hoover, Commentary on "The Nurse's Appeal to Conscience" in *Cases in Bioethics: Selections from the Hastings Center Report*, 3rd ed. ed. Bette-Jane Crigger (New York: St. Martin's Press, 1998).

15. Mila Ann Aroskar, Commentary on "The Nurse's Appeal to Conscience" in *Cases in Bioethics Selections from the Hastings Center Report*, 3rd ed. ed. Bette-Jane Crigger (New York: St. Martin's Press, 1998).

Chapter 15

Multicultural Perspectives in Health Care

More and more it is being recognized that some principles of American health care ethics may not be universally accepted. For example, Western health care ethics "endorses certain practices such as informed consent, disclosure of diagnosis and prognosis, and termination of treatment under certain conditions of terminal illness" (1). These practices, in turn, "reflect certain values widely held in Western culture: the autonomy of the individual person, the imperatives favoring truthfulness and open communication, and the realistic assessment of the efficacy of medical care" (1). However, health care workers who are trained in these practices and values may encounter patients and families from various cultures and subcultures who "react negatively or paradoxically to these practices" (1). In such cases, conflicts can arise between health care providers and patients and their families.

225

In this chapter you will learn about:

- The practice of telling the truth about her condition to a patient who is terminally ill;
- Cultures with different views than American bioethics on truth telling to the terminally ill, patient autonomy, pain management, and the practice of informed consent;
- Ways in which health care providers can deal with multiculturalism;
- The competing theories of ethical relativism and ethical objectivism.

Case Study

The Pleasant Hill Care Center is located in a Midwestern community that has recently seen an influx of Asian residents. This is because of a faculty and student exchange program established by a local college.

Mr. Chang has come with his family to the United States from China to teach at the college. Mr. Chang's mother, 84, accompanied them to the United States because she is a widow and in poor health. In fact, multiple health problems and general physical debilitation soon led to her placement in the Pleasant Hill Care Center.

The adjustment to the nursing home has been very difficult for Mrs. Chang, in part because she speaks very little English. Her son and daughter-in-law usually serve as interpreters for communications with the staff, but there are also some Chinese students from the college who visit the nursing home to converse with her.

Mrs. Chang becomes increasingly listless, and spends much of her time sleeping. When blood is discovered in her stools, she is sent to the hospital for diagnostic tests. The tests indicate that she has colon cancer, which has rapidly spread to other parts of her body. An oncologist, Dr. Marilyn Scott, tells her son that the cancer is "too far gone" for chemotherapy or surgery to be viable treatments. Dr. Scott recommends that measures be taken simply to keep her as comfortable as possible until she dies, most likely in just a few months.

Dr. Scott asks Mr. Chang how his mother should be approached with this bad news. Mr. Chang insists that his mother be told absolutely nothing about her condition. He himself does not plan to tell her anything, and he virtually threatens Dr. Scott not to discuss anything with his mother through another interpreter.

Dr. Scott thinks that Mr. Chang's reaction comes from the initial shock of learning that his mother has a terminal illness. So she asks a physician assistant, Bob Merrill, to approach Mr. Chang again in a few days. However, Mr. Chang reacts to Mr. Merrill in precisely the same way. A week goes by and Mr. Merrill tries having another conversation with Mr. Chang but he remains adamant in his position.

Dr. Scott thinks that Mrs. Chang could profit from the hospice program available at the nursing home, but her son would not even listen to information about it. Dr. Scott also feels that a do-not-resuscitate order should be discussed with her.

Both Dr. Scott and Mr. Merrill believe strongly that Mr. Chang is being unfair to his mother in not allowing her to be informed of her condition. After all, it is her life and it should be up to her to decide what treatments she does and does not want. Indeed, Dr. Scott has such negative feelings about the way in which Mr. Chang wants to handle the situation and his absolute refusal to agree to "standard medical practice" that she considers withdrawing from the case entirely.

Truth Telling to the Terminally Ill

The case of Mrs. Chang concerns the ethical issue of telling the truth about a terminal condition to a patient. Both the physician and physician assistant involved in her care are concerned that she does not know her diagnosis and hence is unable to make her own decisions about the type and extent of treatment to receive as her life draws to a close. These concerns on the part of health care providers reflect two principles of American health care ethics: truth telling to the terminally ill and patient autonomy.

Within American health care a distinct change in attitude has taken place concerning truth telling to the terminally ill. Prior to 1960, the predominant practice was to withhold information from the patient, for fear that frank truth would frighten or harm her (2). Studies indicate that, in 1960, about 90 percent of cancer physicians favored nondisclosure of the diagnosis. But 20 years later, 90 percent favored disclosure of the diagnostic information to patients (2).

In fact, the *Ethical and Religious Directives for Catholic Health Care Services* in the United States make truth telling to the terminally ill a matter of policy:

Persons in danger of death should be provided with whatever information is necessary to help them understand their condition and have the opportunity to discuss their condition with their family members and care providers. They should be offered the appropriate medical information that would make it possible to address the morally legitimate choices available to them. (3)

Various concerns have been expressed about a policy of telling the truth to patients who are terminally ill. For one thing, medical diagnoses and prognoses are never 100 percent certain. We can all think of cases in which someone was expected to die but unexpectedly recovered. So why cause a patient distress unnecessarily? Others have questioned the ability of patients who are debilitated by a serious illness to understand the information given to them and whether patients in fact want bad news communicated to them. Further, there is concern that announcement of a terminal illness may harm the patient by causing fright or depression, by causing her to cease to struggle against the disease, or even by prompting a cardiac arrest or suicide (4).

On the other hand, it has been argued that patients often intuitively have a sense of their condition. As Kübler-Ross indicates from her studies with the dying: "When we asked our patients how they had been told, we learned that all the patients know about their terminal illness anyway, whether they were explicitly told or not . . . " (5). Indeed, patients can be relieved when the issue of their terminal condition is brought out into the open. Proponents of truth telling also call attention to studies that indicate that a large majority of persons say they would like to be told of the diagnosis of a serious illness (4). And it is pointed out that a policy of truth telling in the case of terminal illness is not equivalent to blurting out medical information coldly. Such a policy can and should be accompanied by "finesse, feeling, warmth, empathy, etc., with regard to how much?—when?—how? . . ." (6).

Finally, while concern has been expressed about possible harmful effects on patients of knowing about terminal illness, it is argued that the withholding of information can also have negative consequences:

> . . . we are also becoming increasingly aware of all that can befall patients in the course of their illness when information is denied or distorted. Lies place them in a position where they no longer participate in choices concerning their own health, including the choice of whether to be a "patient" in the first place. A terminally ill person who is not informed that his illness is incurable and that he is near death cannot make decisions about the end of his life; about whether or not to enter a hospital, or to have surgery; where and with whom to spend his last days; how to put his affairs in order—these most personal choices cannot be made if he is kept in the dark, or given contradictory hints and clues. (4)

Positively stated, truth telling to terminally ill patients may allow them to participate in decisions about their medical treatment, to make more satisfying use of the time remaining to them, and to make preparations for death. And this is where there is a connection between truth telling to the terminally ill and patient autonomy. It is argued that patients should be told the truth about their terminal condition precisely so that they themselves can make choices about and direct what happens at the end of their lives.

To someone imbued with the principles of truth telling and autonomy (as were the physician and physician assistant involved in the care of Mrs. Chang), it might appear that Mrs. Chang's family is not acting in her best interests. A conflict arises in the case of Mrs. Chang precisely because her family is from a culture that brings a different set of beliefs and values to bear in caring for the terminally ill. Many Chinese believe that a person is entitled to be treated as a child when ill, deserving protection. To tell someone that he or she is dying is considered to be not only rude but dangerous, like casting a death curse upon the person that will make the person despair and die even sooner. Thus discussions of code status or the possibility of hospice care are precluded. Further, it is believed that truth telling about a terminal illness signifies the withdrawal of hope, indicating to patients that their health care providers have given up on them and that they might as well "give up" too. While a family may be fully aware of the grave diagnosis, cultural expectations are that they will not acknowledge or discuss it openly (7).

This is a very different mindset from current Western health care practice in which truth telling is seen positively as something that enables the patient to have some control over the end of her life. Nevertheless, knowledge of this cultural background makes the behavior of Mr. Chang understandable.

How can health care workers identify when a conflict situation with a patient and her family is due to cultural differences? They can try to learn as much as possible about the cultural beliefs and practices of ethnic groups with whom they have contact (8). To do this, they might "identify one or two individuals from the patient's family or community who are willing to act as cultural informants" (8). Or they might "consult with other health care practitioners from the same ethnic group as the patient" (8). Or again, they might call on the resources of local colleges and universities (8).

How can health care workers *resolve conflicts* due to cultural differences? In such cases health care workers need to be flexible; they need to show respect for beliefs and practices different than their own; and they need to be willing to compromise (8). For example, in the case of Mrs. Chang and her family, an accommodation might be achieved between American and Chinese values by her health care providers asking Mrs. Chang if she has any questions about her condition or treatment, and by assuring her family that she will not be told any more than she wishes to know (8). Ethically, these accommodations to persons of different cultures respect their right to self-determination and autonomy (8).

Further Examples of Cultural Diversity

Autonomy is a prominent value in contemporary American health care ethics. In the context of end-of-life decision making, the emphasis on autonomy has been described in this way:

> Traditionally, bioethics theory and practice have relied heavily on the Western philosophical principle of respect for persons to justify a model of end-of-life decision making that is focused on the rights and wishes of the individual patient. An important goal of bioethics innovation— such as advance care directives and open disclosure of prognosis—is to promote control of medical decision making at the end of life by an autonomous, fully informed patient.
>
> In the United States, the "ideal" patient is a self-governing individual who is future oriented and willing to engage in frank discussions about difficult medical topics, including planning for his or her own death. (9)

However, "some have argued that this preoccupation with individual rights to the exclusion of other values," such as family integrity and the responsibility of health care professionals, "may reflect a cultural bias on the part of the Western medical and bioethics communities" (10). It has been suggested that "the notion of an informed active decision maker may not be a universally held ideal of the good patient but rather, a very specific set of values based on a particular Western philosophical tradition" (9).

For example, Latinos tend to be group-oriented and family-oriented rather than individualistic (11). For this reason, health issues are dealt with at the family level (11).

> . . . giving consent for a diagnostic or surgical procedure is a family affair for most Latinos. Before making a final decision, adults often insist on holding family meetings to seek the advice and opinions of other adult family members, usually brothers, sisters, and even *comadres* ("co-mothers," closest female friends) and *compadres* (male equivalent of co-madres). . . . Adult family members are generally responsible for giving

consent to carry out a procedure for a spouse, a child, or an elderly person. . . .

Adult children are traditionally responsible for elderly adults, who tend to voluntarily abdicate responsibility for their own health care and well-being. An elderly Latino or Latina very rarely makes major decisions regarding health issues. If consent is requested for a diagnostic or surgical procedure, elderly Latinos will often tell you that the decision is in the hands of their family. Often, brothers and sisters, children, and even grandchildren convene at an urgent family meeting to discuss the issue and adults take a vote. If one relative lives out of town or in another country, the meeting (and therefore the procedure) may be postponed for a later date to await the arrival of that person. (11)

It has also been noted that "in many Asian societies, ideas about 'selfhood' vary from the Western ideal of an autonomous individual" so that a "sociocentric or relational sense of self often leads to decision-making styles at odds with Western bioethics ideals" (12).

Another area of cross-cultural difference is pain management. American palliative care specialists emphasize controlling a patient's pain, even to the point of putting patients into a state of diminished consciousness or continuing unconsciousness until death naturally occurs (see Chapter 11). On the other hand, "mindfulness and mental clarity are important values for Buddhists," as evidenced by the importance placed on meditation (13). Buddhism emphasizes "the importance of death with an unclouded mind wherever possible" (13). Hence some Buddhists may be "unwilling to take pain-relieving drugs or strong sedatives, and even those who are not in a terminal condition might prefer to remain as alert as possible, rather than take analgesics that would impair their mental or sensory capacities" (13).

Or again, it is commonplace in the United States to have individuals sign a written consent form for a variety of diagnostic tests and medical procedures. However, an Arab who has verbally agreed to a test or procedure may become irate when subsequently asked to sign a written consent form and may refuse to do so (1). This is because Arabs regard a verbal agreement as "binding and equal to their written agreement" (1). To press them further for a written agreement "only suggests mistrust of their verbal contract" and challenges their personal honor (1).

What does this cultural diversity mean for ethics and the validity of ethical principles and judgments? Can we ever say for sure that anything is ethically right or wrong?

Ethical Relativism Versus Ethical Objectivism

Multiculturalism in health care raises the question of *ethical objectivism* versus *ethical relativism.* Ethical objectivists maintain that there are some basic ethical standards and values that hold for everyone everywhere. An ethical relativist, on the other hand, denies this and maintains that what is right and wrong varies among different cultures and groups. So, for example, an ethical relativist might maintain that polygamy (the practice of having more than one wife at the same time) is ethically wrong in one country but ethically permissible in another. The ethical relativist does *not* maintain merely that people in the two countries may *think* polygamy is wrong (or right), but that polygamy is *in fact* wrong in one country but right in another (see Chapter 1).

That different cultural groups consider different actions to be ethically right and wrong is often presented as evidence in favor of ethical relativism. For example, Americans favor telling the complete and absolute truth about terminal illness to a patient, whereas (as we have seen) this is considered the wrong thing to do by the Chinese. But does this really mean there are no shared ethical principles among all human beings? Those favoring ethical objectivism argue that different cultures and groups may share the same basic ethical principles and values but may put these principles and values into practice in different ways because of different circumstances or a different set of factual beliefs (see Chapter 1). For example, in the case of an Arab agreeing to a medical test or procedure, the basic point of giving consent is really not at issue; the question concerns the way giving consent is practiced. Americans emphasize written consent, whereas Arabs place a high value on verbal consent. In the case of Mrs. Chang, we learn that the Chinese place a high priority on protecting patients from harm. American health care ethicists adhere to the principle of nonmaleficence, recognizing an obligation of health care workers to "do no harm" to patients (see Chapter 1). The same basic value is held in the two cultures and the dispute arises over the consequences believed to follow from truth telling in the case of terminal illness. The Chinese see truth telling as harming the patient by causing her to lose hope and bringing on an earlier death. Americans, on the other hand, have questioned whether these bad effects really come about for most patients and see harm to the patient coming from withholding the truth about terminal illness. If the Chinese and the Americans could be brought to agree factually on the consequences of truth telling in the case of terminal illness, they might well agree ethically on whether this should be done.

CHAPTER SUMMARY

Key Terms and Concepts

principle of patient autonomy: self-determination; an individual's right to hold views, make choices, and take actions based on personal values and beliefs.

ethical objectivism: the position that there are some basic ethical principles that hold for everyone everywhere.

ethical relativism: the position that what is in fact right and wrong varies among different cultures and societies.

Key Points

- Telling a terminally ill patient the truth about her condition is now a standard practice in American health care. This is done to allow a patient to participate in decisions about medical treatments, to make more satisfying use of the time remaining to her, and to make appropriate preparations for death. In other words, truth telling is supposed to enable a patient to better direct and control what happens at the end of her life and thus follows from the ethical principle of patient autonomy.

- Not all cultures and societies favor telling the truth to a patient who is terminally ill because they regard it as harming the patient.

- American culture emphasizes individual autonomy in health care decision making, whereas other cultures favor a family model of decision making.

- American palliative care practices emphasize controlling pain, even at the cost of putting the patient into a state of diminished consciousness or continuing unconsciousness until death occurs. However, a person from another cultural tradition may value mental lucidity over pain control.

- American health care has adopted a procedure of requiring written consent from the patient or his proxy. Other cultures may not have the same emphasis and, for example, may attach more importance to verbal assent than does American culture.

- When health care providers are involved in a conflict situation with a patient and/or his family due to cultural differences, they should try to learn about the beliefs and practices of the patient and his family, be flexible, and seek courses of action that can accommodate the cultural beliefs and practices of the patient and his family.

■ The fact that beliefs and practices may differ among various cultures and societies does *not* necessarily mean that human beings cannot agree on what is ethically right and wrong and have no shared ethical principles and values. Various cultures and societies may share basic ethical values and principles, but put them into practice in different ways because of different circumstances or factual beliefs.

FOR FURTHER DISCUSSION

1. What ethnic and racial groups are present in your geographical area? How much do you know about their beliefs and practices regarding the provision of health care? Where or from whom can you find out more information?
2. Reflect on your own cultural background and how your extended family approaches health care. Do you see any differences from what is considered "standard practice" in American health care?
3. You are working with Pedro Garcia to help him stop smoking. To motivate him, you repeatedly tell him about the harmful effects smoking will have on his own health. However, he is not responding to these warnings. Given that Latinos tend to be group-oriented and family-oriented rather than individualistic, would another kind of message be more effective in motivating him to stop smoking? (11)
4. Do you see any value in a family model of health care decision making in contrast to individual autonomy? Any drawbacks?

References

1. Afaf Ibrahim Meleis and Albert R. Jonsen, "Ethical Crises and Cultural Differences," *The Western Journal of Medicine* 138/6 (June 1983): 889–93.
2. Howard Brody, "The Physician/Patient Relationship," in *Medical Ethics*, ed. Robert M. Veatch (Boston, MA: Jones and Bartlett, 1989).
3. United States Conference of Catholic Bishops, *Ethical and Religious Directives for Catholic Health Care Services*, 5th ed. (2009), no. 55. http://www.usccb .org. Accessed March 2016.
4. Sissela Bok, "Lies to the Sick and Dying," in *Lying: Moral Choice in Public and Private Life* (New York, NY: Pantheon, 1978).
5. Elisabeth Kübler-Ross, *On Death and Dying* (New York: Macmillan, 1969).

6. Orville N. Griese, *Catholic Identity in Health Care: Principles and Practice* (Braintree: MA: Pope John Center, 1987).

7. Jessica H. Muller and Brian Desmond, "Ethical Dilemmas in a Cross-cultural Context, A Chinese Example," *The Western Journal of Medicine* 157/3 (September 1992): 323–27.

8. Robert D. Orr, Patricia A. Marshall, and Jamie Osborn, "Cross-cultural Considerations in Clinical Ethics Consultations," *Archives of Family Medicine* 4 (February 1995): 159–64.

9. Patricia A. Marshall, Barbara A. Koenig, Donelle M. Barnes, and Anne J. Davis, "Multiculturalism, Bioethics, and End-of-Life Care: Case Narratives of Latino Cancer Patients," in *Health Care Ethics: Critical Issues for the 21st Century*, eds. John F. Monagle and David C. Thomasma (Gaithersburg, MD: Aspen, 1998).

10. Leslie J. Blackhall, Sheila T. Murphy, Gelya Frank, Vicki Michel, and Stanley Azen, "Ethnicity and Attitudes Toward Patient Autonomy," *Journal of the American Medical Association* 274/10 (September 13, 1995): 820–25.

11. Nilda Chong, *The Latino Patient A Cultural Guide for Health Care Providers* (Yarmouth, ME: Intercultural Press, 2002).

12. Barbara A. Koenig and Jan Gates-Williams, "Understanding Cultural Difference in Caring for Dying Patients," *Western Journal of Medicine* 163/3 (September 1995): 244–49.

13. Damien Keown, "End of Life: the Buddhist View," *The Lancet* 366 (September 10, 2005): 952–55.

Part Four
Special Topics

Chapter 16

Issues in Organ Procurement and Allocation

When obtaining or renewing a driver's license, you may be asked if you wish to be an organ donor if death should occur. This is one of the measures being used to try to increase the number of organ donors since many more patients are in need of organ transplants at any given time than the number of organs actually available for transplant (1). This fact of a discrepancy between patient need and available resources raises yet another issue. Once an organ becomes available for transplant, how do we fairly decide who should receive it? This is a particularly weighty question because, in making the allocation decision, we may literally be deciding who lives and who dies (2).

In this chapter you will learn about:

■ Standards for determining death and the relation of these standards to organ procurement;

- Actual and proposed ways of recruiting organ donors;
- Criteria and principles for deciding on the distribution of organs to particular patients.

Case Study

Berta Romero has worked as a respiratory therapist at Lakeland Community Hospital for 10 years. She has been involved in removing ventilators from dying patients on many occasions. However, an incident occurred recently, which left her feeling "shaken."

Berta was paged to come to a room near the hospital's surgery center. In it she found a patient on a ventilator. She was told that the patient was dying and had been moved to this room from the intensive care unit (ICU). The ventilator would be removed and, as soon as the patient's heart stopped, the patient would be taken into surgery to remove organs for transplantation purposes.

Berta has always been an advocate of organ donation. However, this procedure makes her feel like a "vulture." Is it right, she wonders, to deliberately choose to let a patient die at a particular time in order that organs can be taken for transplantation to others?

■ ■ ■

Determining Death and Organ Procurement

Living persons can donate some organs and tissues—such as kidneys, a segment of the liver, a lobe of the lung, and portions of the intestine and pancreas (3). From an ethical point of view, a living donor can "give organs whose removal will not adversely affect his or her ability to live in a relatively healthy state" (4).

All organs and tissues that can be transplanted can be obtained from those who are deceased (4). In the latter case, the *dead donor rule* is currently followed; that is, organs cannot be taken for transplant purposes until the patient has reliably been pronounced dead (4). Thus the practice of organ transplantation leads us into the question of the definition and determination of death.

Today, two different standards for determining death are widely accepted. An individual may be declared dead who has sustained *either* the irreversible cessation of circulatory and respiratory functions *or* the irreversible cessation of all functions of the entire brain, including the brainstem ("whole brain death"). (4) The first is a cardiopulmonary criterion of death, and the second, a neurological criterion (4).

Concomitantly, there are two types of organ donation. In donation after death by neurologic criteria (brain death), the donor is brought to the operating room on a ventilator and organ procurement occurs in the operating room while the patient remains intubated with a beating heart (5). In donation after cardiac death, a decision is first made to discontinue ventilation or other life-sustaining treatments for a patient who is expected to die quickly after cessation of life support; then the patient may be extubated in the area of the operating room to minimize the time between death and organ procurement (5).

In the case scenario involving respiratory therapist Berta Romero, the patient's organs would be retrieved for transplant purposes after the patient's heart stopped beating. Special problems are posed in using such non-heart-beating donors:

> A key challenge to procuring organs from non-heart-beating cadavers is posed by warm ischemic damage, caused by the lack of blood perfusion while the organs are still in the body of the newly deceased donor. To prevent or limit this damage, the time between the cessation of circulation ("effective asystole") and the procurement of organs must be minimized. For this purpose, the final cardiac contractions must be *controlled*: In the moments following asystole, the body must be prepared for surgeons either to remove the organs promptly or to maintain their viability for transplantation in the ensuing hours. For the moment of cardiac arrest to be controlled in this way, the prospective organ donor must be a patient from whom a ventilator and perhaps other forms of life-sustaining treatment will be withdrawn, either in accordance with the patient's wishes or the wishes of a surrogate. In other words, a potential non-heart-beating donor, in the vast majority of cases, is an individual who is ventilator-dependent but not yet deceased according to today's neurological standard. The ventilator is then removed, the patient is watched and kept comfortable until the heart stops circulating blood through the body, a waiting period is observed (usually two to five minutes), and then the surgical procurement of organs begins. (4)

The practice of *controlled donation after cardiac death* raises various questions. Following the dead donor rule, can we be sure that the patient is in fact dead when the procedure of organ retrieval is begun? How long should we wait after the patient's heart has stopped before the retrieval procedure is started? Could the patient have been resuscitated and brought back to life? To secure an organ for transplant, will life-sustaining treatment (such as a ventilator) be withdrawn too soon? Overall, will good quality end-of-life care be compromised for the patient–donor? (4).

Thus it has been proposed that "a morally sound hospital policy" on planned donation after cardiac death should include the following stipulations (6):

- The decision to withdraw medical interventions must be made independently of the decision to donate an organ.
- Organ donors must receive the same end-of-life palliative care as non-donors.
- The hospital should provide the donor's family with the option of being present when life support is withdrawn and, in general, take every measure to permit family and friends to say goodbye in a dignified way.
- Procurement teams must wait the recommended amount of time after the permanent cessation of heart function before beginning the removal of organs.
- The medical staff overseeing withdrawal of medical interventions must not hasten the patient's death, even if the organs might become unusable for transplantation.
- If patients do not die quickly enough to become donors, they should be returned to the intensive care unit to die in a peaceful and respectful way (6).

Incorporating such stipulations into hospital policy on organ retrieval should work against a view of planned donation after cardiac death as nothing more than "letting patients die so that their organs can be used for transplant."

Recruiting Organ Donors

The United States currently operates under a system of *altruistic donation* of organs and tissues. Individuals (or their family or proxy decision maker) must voluntarily make the choice to donate organs and tissues, without compensation. However, under the current system of altruistic donation there is a serious shortage of needed organs (7). Some contend that the "current altruistic system has not failed as much as it has not been fully promoted" in that many potential donor families are simply never asked about donating the organs of their deceased relative (7). At the same time, various alternative programs have been proposed to increase organ donation.

One proposal is to provide *financial incentives* for organ donation. For example, an individual might agree in advance to donate organs upon death, with payment to beneficiaries or to his estate occurring after donation has taken place (7). Or again, organ donation might be accompanied by a set reimbursement for funeral expenses (7), or tax credits might be provided to the donor or to his family (8). If a system of financial incentives increases the supply of organs, such incentives would be justified by the saving of lives that would otherwise be lost (7). Further, it is argued that "some form of compensation is the right thing to do" because, at present, "the donor and the family are the only participants not directly benefitting from the process" of organ donation (7).

From an ethical point of view, there is a concern that providing financial incentives for organ donation may lead to decreased respect for life and the sanctity of the human body (7), with the human body becoming "a commodity to be bought, sold and bartered for in a manner similar to any other good or service" (7). There is also a danger that financial incentives for organ donation could coerce the poor into agreeing to donate their organs (7). Moreover, there is a fear that a system of financial reimbursement for organ donation would create an atmosphere in society downgrading the virtue of altruism (9).

An alternative proposal is granting *preferred status* for organ donors. In other words, "individuals who have signified their intention to be organ/tissue donors … would receive points or other value that would somewhat facilitate the likelihood of receiving an organ, should they need it in the future" (10). This benefit might also extend to "first degree relatives of those who have signed up or have actually been donors" (10). An argument in favor of granting preferred status is based on justice. Specifically, "is it fair for an individual who is willing to participate in the system of transplantation to not receive an organ while another medically similar individual who was unwilling to participate receives a transplant?" (10). Further, unlike providing financial incentives for organ donation, preferred status is equitable across economic strata of society; the value of a life-giving organ is the same to a very poor disadvantaged person as to someone who is wealthy (10). At the same time, there are practical difficulties in determining fairly the weight to be given to the intention to be an organ donor (10). For example, it might be a tie-breaker, other things being equal (10), but it "should probably not be sufficient to place an elective case with a short time on the list ahead of one who is about to die, or who has been waiting for years" (10).

Another possible approach to organ donation is *presumed consent.* Under this system, a "candidate for cadaveric organ and tissue recovery is presumed to have consented to organ and tissue recovery if he or she has not registered a refusal" (11). This approach is grounded on our duty to promote the good of society (11).

> The communitarian view holds that individuals have a moral duty to help others when the cost to the individual of helping is very low. Since cadaveric organ donation can save the lives of others and causes no significant harm to the decedent or the family, individuals who do not object on religious grounds have a moral duty to donate their organs. (12)

At the same time, this approach respects individual autonomy "by giving objectors to organ donation an opportunity to empower their anti-donation preference" (11). Further, presumed consent would eliminate the need to ask the donor's family for consent at a time when the family is grieving (11). Concerns about presumed consent focus on the practical difficulties of ensuring that all who object to organ donation in fact have the opportunity to register their refusal with public authorities and setting up the mechanisms for registering and transmitting objection status (11).

Yet another proposal for increasing organ donation is known as *required response* or *mandated choice* (11, 12). Under this system, all adults would be required by public authorities to express their preferences regarding organ donation (i.e., their willingness to donate or objection to donation) when, for example, they renew their driver's licenses, file income tax forms, or perform some other task mandated by the state (11, 12). These preferences would be recorded in a national donor registry (11). This approach is supported by research indicating that the primary reason people do not sign organ donor cards is because of the fact that no authority has asked them (11). From an ethical point of view, this approach respects the value of individual autonomy as all adult persons make a decision for or against organ donation (11).

Case Study

Allen Potter is a lab technician at Mercy Medical Center. He has been asked to do three lab tests—bilirubin, international normalized ratio (INR), and creatinine—for Sam Langan in preparation for placing him on the waiting list for a liver transplant (13).

Sam is 68, and a prominent attorney in the community. He is still active in his church, and has served several terms on the school board. He is currently chair of the annual United Way fund drive. However, throughout his life Sam has struggled with the problem of heavy drinking, which is the reason he needs a liver transplant. Two years ago he voluntarily entered a rehab program, and has had his drinking under control since that time.

Allen Potter has no doubt in his mind that Sam is "worthy" of a liver transplant. He has been, and continues to be, a valuable member of the community. Allen has heard stories of some people waiting for years to get an organ, while others seem to get them almost immediately. Allen hopes Sam can get a transplant before he becomes too debilitated, or even dies.

■ ■ ■

Once organs or tissues are available for transplant, the question must be faced of who should receive them since there are many more people in need of transplants than there are organs and tissues available. This is the issue to which we now turn.

Allocating Organs to Transplant Recipients

Developing a method for allocating organs among possible recipients is a work in progress. Changes and refinements in procedures are ongoing. We will describe various allocation procedures that have been used.

In the case of living organ donors, donation may be *directed* or *nondirected*. In directed donation, the organ donor specifies the recipient of the organ. For example, blood relatives of the transplant candidate, such as parents, brothers or sisters, or adult children, may engage in directed donation. Directed donation may also be used by persons who have some type of personal or social connection with the transplant candidate, such as a spouse or significant other, a friend, or a coworker. Even strangers who have learned about the transplant candidate may engage in directed donation. On the other hand, nondirected donation occurs when individuals donate to an unspecified, anonymous candidate on the transplant waiting list (3).

A particular type of directed donation is *paired donation* or *paired exchange*. This arrangement involves two pairs, e.g., of living kidney donors and transplant candidates who have incompatible blood types, with the two transplant candidates "trading" donors with blood types compatible to them (3). This arrangement is easiest to understand through an example:

> Barbara wants to donate to her sister Donna, but they do not have matching blood types. Carlos wants to donate to his wife Maria, but they are also not compatible. By "swapping" donors so that Carlos matches Donna and Barbara matches Maria, two transplants are made possible. (3)

This type of arrangement can also involve multiple living donor and transplant candidate pairs. (3)

Yet another arrangement available to living donors is *donor waiting list exchange*. For example, a living donor who has an incompatible blood type with the intended kidney transplant candidate will donate to an anonymous candidate on the waiting list, with the intended transplant candidate in turn moving up on the waiting list (14).

In the case of directed donation to a relative by blood or marriage or to a significant other, the practice of directed donation can be justified ethically by appealing to the intuition that we have stronger obligations to persons with whom we are in special relationships than to strangers (15). The practice of directed donation can also be justified on utilitarian grounds (see Chapter 1); namely, that it makes more organs available for transplant and hence saves additional lives (assuming that the donor would not be inclined to donate to an anonymous recipient). What has been ethically controversial, however, is the direction of organs to a specific social group; for example, to a group defined by race, religion, ethnicity, gender, or sexual orientation (15). In one recorded case, a man who was a sympathizer of the Ku Klux Klan was shot and killed in a robbery. His family agreed to donate his organs, but stipulated "donation to White recipients only" (15). Directed donation to a particular social group has been opposed on the grounds that it represents "unequal treatment based on morally irrelevant considerations" (15).

The case study involving Sam Langan concerns transplant of a liver most probably to be obtained from a cadaver. At one point, the United Network for Organ Sharing (UNOS) adopted the principle that donated livers should go to the patient most urgently in need at the time that a transplantable liver becomes available (13). Specifically, the following procedure was developed for making allocation decisions for individuals aged 12 or older:

- Status 1 patients are those who have acute (sudden and severe onset) liver failure and a life expectancy of hours to a few days without a transplant.
- Other candidates for liver transplants are given a score between 6 (less ill) and 40 (gravely ill) based on how urgently the candidate needs a transplant within the next 3 months, as calculated by a formula using three lab test results.
- If the donor is younger than 18, then the following prioritization scheme is used:
  — The liver is given first to a Status 1 patient.
  — The liver is offered next to candidates age 11 or younger in the geographical region.
  — The liver is then made available to candidates with a score of 15 or higher, locally and then regionally, with patients aged 12–17 considered ahead of adult patients.
- If the donor is 18 or older, then the following prioritization scheme is used:
  — The liver is given first to Status 1 candidates, locally and regionally.

— The liver is offered next to candidates with a score of 15 or higher, locally and then regionally.

— The liver is then made available to candidates with a score of 14 or less, locally and then regionally.

— Finally, the liver is made available to any compatible candidates nationwide, beginning with Status 1 candidates and then to those with the highest scores.

■ The time of a transplant candidate on the waiting list is considered only when there are two or more transplant candidates with the same blood type and score (13).

In sum, the criteria used for allocating livers for transplant purposes include urgency of need, age, geographical location, and time on the transplant waiting list.

UNOS has used somewhat different criteria for allocating other types of organs. In the case of lung transplants, the patient's "score" has been "an estimate of the severity of each candidate's illness and his or her chance of success following a lung transplant" (16). In 2014 a revised set of criteria went into effect for allocating kidneys, which provide that "people who are expected to need a kidney for the longest time will be matched more often with kidneys that have the longest expected function" (17). The revised criteria also provide that "groups of people who are hard to match with kidneys, based on their blood type or immune sensitivity, will also get additional priority" (17).

From an ethical point of view, the allocation of organs has been described in terms of balancing two values: *efficiency* in the use of organs and *fairness* in distribution (i.e., justice or equity) (18). From a justice perspective, concern has been raised about the use of geographical criteria for allocating organs.

The aforementioned scheme for allocating liver transplants contains stipulations prioritizing allocation at local, regional, and national levels. In defense of granting priority at the local level, it may be argued that such prioritization will make people more willing to donate organs because "it is natural for each community to feel it should serve its own members first" and because people "like to think that they are helping their neighbors" (15). It may also be argued that granting priority at the local level helps maintain the quality of organs by keeping ischemia times brief, and further, that it supports local transplant centers that enable patients to be transplanted close to home (15). On the other hand, geographical prioritization at local and regional levels may entail the inequity of "directing organs to healthier patients over those who are desperately ill simply because of the morally irrelevant variable of where one happens to live"

(15). Or again, such geographical prioritization may result in unequal waiting times for an organ for patients with equal severity of illness (15). Such inequities are brought forward as reasons for establishing a single *national* list for organ transplantation (15). The only recognized exception in which organs could be "restricted solely on the basis of geographical proximity between the donor and the recipient" would be "those cases in which medical necessity prohibits transport of the organ in a way that would maintain viability" (15).

In our case study the transplant candidate, Sam Langan, is 68 years old. Should his age be a factor in prioritizing him for a liver transplant? Intuitively, we may well feel that an 80-year-old should not have the same priority for an organ transplant as someone who is 20, or 30, or 40 years old. But what about someone who is 68?

Ethicists have proposed different positions on the appropriateness of considering age as one factor figuring into allocation of organs for transplant. One view is that "the elderly deserve equal treatment" with other candidates (15). The reason is that "justice requires treating similarly situated people equally and that those who are sickest deserve priority even if it is not always the most efficient use of resources" (15). Thus "all persons who are equally sick, regardless of age, deserve equal treatment" (15). A contrasting view works with the concept of *justice-over-a-lifetime*:

> It asks who is worst off considering people's whole lives. From the moment-in-time perspective, a 40-year-old and a 70-year-old dying of heart failure are equally poor off, but considering their entire lives who could deny that the one who was healthy enough to make it to 70 is much better off? To be fair, we need to allocate our resources so that the 40-year-old has a chance to make it to 70. From this over-a-lifetime perspective, justice requires that we target organs for these younger persons who are so poorly off that they will not make it to old age without being given special priority. The younger the age of the person needing an organ, the higher the claim. (15)

In other words, on this scheme entitlement to organs would be inversely proportional to age, and this factor would apply regardless of where one is in the life span (15). Further, this standard "would provide a smooth, gradual priority inversely related to age rather than producing a precipitous drop off in entitlement at some birthday" (15). Thus, applied to the case of someone like Sam Langan at age 68, the justice-over-a-lifetime standard would take his age into account as a factor lessening his entitlement to a transplant without totally precluding the possibility of an organ transplant for him.

In the case study Sam Langan's need for a liver transplant has been caused by heavy drinking. Behaviors such as drinking alcohol, smoking cigarettes, eating fatty foods, and a failure to exercise increase the likelihood of needing an organ transplant (15). Ethically, the question has been raised of whether persons engaging in such behaviors have less claim to an organ transplant in a prioritization scheme, or even whether they should be totally excluded from eligibility. Before giving an affirmative answer to this question, it is critical to determine the extent to which such behaviors are voluntary and the extent to which genetic, psychological, and economic factors play a causal role (15). However, this is not an easy task and the answer is not clear cut. The Ethics and Social Impact Committee of the Transplant and Health Policy Center in Ann Arbor, Michigan, has argued that, even if alcoholism involves an ethically blameworthy weakness of will, it is not legitimate to categorically deny liver transplants to alcoholics suffering from end-stage cirrhosis (19). They point out that, as a general rule, we do not engage in moral evaluation of transplant candidates as a condition for eligibility: "We do not seek to determine whether a particular transplant candidate is an abusive parent or a dutiful daughter, whether candidates cheat on their income taxes or their spouses, or whether potential recipients pay their parking tickets or routinely lie when they think it is in their best interests" (19). Similarly, an alcoholic should not be subjected to personal moral scrutiny as a condition for receiving an organ transplant.

In the case scenario the lab technician Allen Potter considers Sam Langan a "worthy" candidate for an organ transplant because of his social contributions. Sam is a prominent attorney, is active in his church, has served several terms on the school board, and is currently chair of the annual United Way fund drive. The rationale for taking into account the social worth of a potential organ recipient might be the following: if a society invests a scarce resource in one person rather than another, society has a right to consider what it will receive in return (20). However, judging someone's social worth in making organ allocation decisions has proven very controversial because of the extremely subjective nature of the judgments involved. Many would not want this to be a factor in allocating organs for transplantation (21).

CHAPTER SUMMARY

Key Terms and Concepts

brain death: the death of a person as determined by the irreversible cessation of all brain functions.

cardiopulmonary death: the death of a person as determined by the irreversible cessation of circulatory and respiratory functions.

controlled donation after cardiac death: a practice of coordinating the withdrawal of life-sustaining treatment with organ retrieval so as to allow prompt retrieval of organs after cardiopulmonary death has occurred.

presumed consent: a candidate for cadaveric organ and tissue recovery is presumed to have consented to organ and tissue recovery if he or she has not registered a refusal.

required response/mandated choice: all adults would be required by public authorities to express their preferences regarding organ donation, either their willingness to donate or objection to donation.

directed organ donation: the organ donor specifies the recipient of the organ.

nondirected organ donation: the donor donates to an unspecified, anonymous candidate on the transplant waiting list.

Key Points

- Living persons can donate some organs and tissues. All organs and tissues that can be transplanted can be obtained from those who are deceased.

- The dead donor rule affirms that, in the case of cadaveric organ and tissue recovery, organs cannot be taken for transplant purposes until the patient has actually been pronounced dead.

- Two different standards are commonly used for determining death: brain death and cardiopulmonary death.

- There are special challenges, medically and ethically, in the case of non-heart-beating organ donation. This practice requires safeguards to be put into place.

- The United States currently operates under a system of *voluntary donation* of organs and tissues. However, this system has left us with an acute shortage of organs for transplantation. Proposed methods for increasing organ donation include offering financial incentives, granting preferred status to receive an organ to those agreeing to donate (or to their families), presuming consent to donate organs, and requiring people to make an explicit choice for or against organ donation. Ethical principles and values are important in evaluating these proposals.

- From an ethical point of view, the allocation of organs has been described in terms of balancing two values: *efficiency* in the use of organs and *fairness* in distribution (i.e., justice or equity).

- There are ethical questions regarding the use of geographical location, age, behavioral responsibility for one's disease, or social worth as criteria in allocating organs for transplantation.

FOR FURTHER DISCUSSION

1. Have you ever been present when someone died? What made you "believe" or "feel" that the person was dead? How do your intuitions about what constitutes death compare with the brain death criterion? With the cardiopulmonary criterion?

2. Have you signed an organ donor card? Why or why not? Share and discuss your responses.

3. Suppose that your sister (or brother), with whom you are quite close, needs a kidney transplant. You are told that you are a good match. You are told that the risks of serious complications following removal of one kidney are rare; the donor's kidney function rapidly returns to approximately 90 percent of what it was before surgery. Nevertheless, should the donor's remaining kidney become diseased or injured later in life, there will be serious consequences for the donor (22).

   ■ *Under these conditions, would you agree to donate one of your kidneys to your sister (or brother)? Why or why not?*

   ■ *Would you feel pressured to donate a kidney by family ties? How do you think your sister (or brother) would react if you declined to donate? How do you think your parents would react if you declined to donate?*

4. Researchers at Ganogen have developed a new technique that may provide more kidneys to people who need such a transplant. A kidney from an aborted human fetus is implanted into a rat where the kidney grows to a larger size. Eventually, kidneys from aborted fetuses could be implanted into larger animals, such as pigs, where the organs could grow large enough to be transplanted into human beings. The researchers have also transplanted human fetal hearts into rats (23). Do you see any ethical issues with what these researchers are doing to provide more organs for human transplant? Can these ethical issues be satisfactorily resolved?

5. In the film *My Sister's Keeper*, Anna is conceived through in vitro fertilization and selected as an embryo that is a genetic match for her sister Kate who suffers from leukemia, so that she can provide compatible organs, blood, and tissue to keep her sister Kate alive (24). Is the course of action taken by the parents regarding Anna permissible from an ethical point of view? (You might want to watch this film.)

6. In the future it may be possible to clone a particular person to provide a compatible source of organs and tissues for transplant purposes (25). Do you think this would be an ethically acceptable use of human cloning?

7. A *xenograft* is the transfer of tissue or organs between individuals of different species. A famous case of cross-species transplantation occurred at Loma Linda University Medical Center when the defective heart of "Baby Fae" was replaced with the heart of a baboon. The infant lived 20 days before rejecting the heart (26). Experimentation with transplantation of animal organs into humans is likely to continue in the future. Do you see any ethical issues with transplanting animal organs into humans?

8. In general, we do not consider social worth as an appropriate criterion to use in making decisions about allocating organs for transplant. However, suppose that a prison inmate, who has been convicted of a serious crime, is in need of an organ transplant. Should the prisoner be considered ineligible for an organ transplant because of his harmful actions against society? How would you feel if the decision was between giving the organ to the prison inmate or to a member of your own family?

References

1. United Network for Organ Sharing, *Transplant Data.* https://www.unos.org/data. Accessed April 2016.

2. National Kidney Foundation, *Organ Donation and Transplantation Statistics.* https://www.kidney.org/news/newsroom/factsheets/Organ-Donation-and-Transplantation-Stats. Accessed April 2016.

3. United Network for Organ Sharing, *Types of Living Donor Transplants.* https://www.unos.org/donation/living-donation. Accessed April 2016.

4. The President's Council on Bioethics, *Controversies on the Determination of Death* (January 2009). https://bioethicsarchive.georgetown.edu/pcbe/reports/death. Accessed April 2016.

5. Dana Lustbader and Michael J. Goldstein, *Fast Facts and Concepts #242 Organ Donation After Cardiac Death.* http://www.mypcnow.org/#!blank/b9ix3. Accessed April 2016.

6. Sam Crowe and Eric Cohen, *Organ Transplantation: Potential Policy Recommendations. A Staff Working Paper of the President's Council on Bioethics.* https://bioethicsarchive.georgetown.edu/pcbe/background/organ-recs.html. Accessed April 2016.

7. Edward W. Nelson, James E. Childress, Jennie Perryman, Victor Robards, Albert Rowan, Michael W. Seely, Sylvester Sterioff, and Mary Rovelli Swanson, *Financial Incentives for Organ Donation. A Report of the Payment Subcommittee, OPTN/UNOS Ethics Committee,* 1993. https://optn.transplant.hrsa.gov/resources/ethics/financial-incentives-for-organ-donation. Accessed April 2016.

8. Arthur L. Caplan, "Organ Procurement: It's Not in the Cards," *Hastings Center Report* 14/5 (October 1984): 9–12.

9. Kathryn Schroeter, "The Ethics of Organ Donation," *Today's O.R. Nurse* (January/February 1995): 8–12.

10. James F. Burdick, Alexander M. Capron, Francis L. Delmonico, Mark D. Ravenscraft, Craig R. Reckhard, and Michael Shapiro, *Preferred Status for Organ Donors. A Report of the OPTN/UNOS Ethics Committee*, 1993. https://optn.transplant.hrsa.gov/resources/ethics/preferred-status-for-organ-donors. Accessed April 2016.

11. J. Michael Dennis, Patricia Hanson, Ernest Hodge, Ruud A.F. Krom, and Robert M. Veatch, *An Evaluation of the Ethics of Presumed Consent and A Proposal Based on Required Response. A Report of the Presumed Consent Subcommittee, OPTN/UNOS Ethics Committee*, 1993. http://optn.transplant.hrsa.gov/resources/ethics/an-evaluation-of-the-ethics-of-presumed-consent. Accessed April 2016.

12. Council on Ethical and Judicial Affairs of the American Medical Association, "Strategies for Cadaveric Organ Procurement," *Journal of the American Medical Association* 272/10 (September 14, 1994): 809–12.

13. United Network for Organ Sharing, *Questions and Answers for Transplant Candidates about MELD and PELD. https://www.unos.org/wp-content/uploads/unos/MELD.PELD*.pdf. Accessed April 2016.

14. UCSF Benioff Children's Hospital, *Kidney Donor Waiting List Exchange.* https://www.ucsfbenioffchildrens.org/programs/kidney-donor-waiting-list-exchange. Accessed April 2016.

15. Robert M. Veatch, *Transplantation Ethics* (Washington, DC: Georgetown University Press, 2000).

16. United Network for Organ Sharing, *Questions and Answers for Transplant Candidates About Lung Allocation.* https://www.unos.org/wp-content/uploads/unos/Lung_Patient.pdf. Accessed April 2016.

17. United Network for Organ Sharing, *Questions and Answers for Transplant Candidates About Kidney Allocation.* https://www.unos.org/wp-content/uploads/unos/Kidney_Brochure.pdf. Accessed April 2016.

18. F. Daniel Davis, *The Ethics of Organ Allocation: Policy Questions Concerning Geography, Age, and Net Benefit. A Staff Discussion Paper of the President's Council on Bioethics*, 2007. https://bioethicsarchive.georgetown.edu/pcbe/background/ethics_of_organ_allocation.html. Accessed April 2016.

19. Carl Cohen, Martin Benjamin, and the Ethics and Social Impact Committee of the Transplant and Health Policy Center, "Alcoholics and Liver Transplantation," *Journal of the American Medical Association* 265 (March 13, 1991): 1299–1301.

20. Nichols Rescher, "The Allocation of Exotic Medical Lifesaving Technology," *Ethics* 79/3 (April 1969): 173–86.

21. *Doctor, I Want …* , Hard Choices Series, KCTS/Seattle, 1980, video.

22. Karen K. Giuliano, "Organ Transplants: Tackling the Tough Ethical Questions," *Nursing* (May 1997): 34–40.

23. Tanya Lewis, *Growing Human Kidneys in Rats Sparks Ethical Debate* (January 21, 2015). http://www.livescience.com/49503-human-kidneys-grown-in-rats.html. Accessed April 2016.

24. Wikipedia, *My Sister's Keeper (film)*. https:/en.wikipedia.org/wiki/My_Sister's_Keeper_film. Accessed April 2016.

25. President's Council on Bioethics, *Human Cloning and Human Dignity* (New York, NY: Public Affairs, 2002).

26. Ricki Lewis, *Human Genetics: Concepts and Applications*, 2nd ed. (Dubuque, IA: Wm C. Brown Publishers, 1997).

Chapter 17

Research and Experimentation Involving Human Subjects

The Nuremberg trials following World War II brought to light medical research and experimentation conducted by the Nazis that was abusive of human subjects. These abuses were prevalent in the concentration camps. At Dachau, for example, "healthy inmates were injected with extracts from the mucous glands of mosquitoes to produce malaria" and then various drugs were "used to determine their relative effectiveness" (1). At Buchenwald, "various kinds of poisons were secretly administered to a number of inmates to test their efficacy" (1). At Ravensbrück, people were deliberately cut and their wounds infected with bacteria in order to test the efficacy of the drug sulfanilamide (1).

Unfortunately, medical experiments abusive of human beings were not limited to Nazi Germany. Questionable research projects have also been conducted within the United States. A prime example is the Tuskegee Syphilis Study conducted under the auspices of the U.S. Department of Public Health:

> From 1932 to 1970, a large but undetermined number of black males suffering from the later stages of syphilis were examined at regular intervals to determine the course their disease was taking. The men in the study were poor and uneducated . . . they were given either no treatment or inadequate treatment, and at least forty of them died as a result of factors connected with their disease. . . . It was known when the study began that those with untreated syphilis have a higher death rate than those whose condition is treated, and although the study was started before the advent of penicillin (which is highly effective against syphilis), other drugs were available but were not used in ways to produce the best results. When penicillin became generally available, it still was not used. (1)

This is not an isolated incident. From the 1940s to the 1960s, chemical testing involving mescaline and LSD was conducted by the American military and intelligence agencies. Experiments took place without the knowledge of the subjects and sometimes resulted in death (2). Also controversial were the Willowbrook hepatitis experiments, which involved mentally challenged children in a state institution as research subjects (1).

Such abusive practices have led to the formulation of *codes of research ethics* such as the *Nuremberg Code* (3), the *Declaration of Helsinki* of the World Medical Association (4), and the Belmont Report (5). Within the United States, health care facilities and research institutes have established institutional review boards (IRBs) to review and approve proposed research projects as a condition for receiving funding from the U.S. Department of Health and Human Services (2).

In this chapter you will learn about:

- General norms and specific criteria used to evaluate proposed research projects;
- Ethical principles underlying these norms and criteria;
- Challenges in obtaining informed consent from potential research subjects;
- Restrictions on proxy consent for participation in research and experimentation.

Case Study

Marilyn Stewart provides occupational therapy services at Sun Valley Care Center. When she makes her visit this week, the administrator calls Marilyn into his office. He tells her that researchers at the state university medical school are conducting a study of a new blood pressure medication using the residents of Sun Valley. This new medication is expected to have fewer of the side effects that many older persons experience with the currently standard medications. However, the administrator points out that "you can never be sure exactly what to expect with medication that is still being tested." He asks Marilyn to watch for unusual symptoms or behavior on the part of residents—which may be a function of the medication—and to alert a nurse on duty about it.

Marilyn notices that the administrator seems quite proud that his facility was chosen by researchers at the state university's medical school to participate in this study. However, she wonders how much the residents understand about the research project in which they are the experimental subjects. Some of the residents are hard of hearing and have poor eyesight. Some suffer from memory loss. Some suffer from dementia, in varying degrees. What kind of explanation of the research study was given to the residents? And how much of the explanation did they understand? Who made the decision that the residents should participate in this research project? Marilyn wonders if the residents of whom she has grown so fond are simply being used as "guinea pigs."

■ ■ ■

Norms and Criteria for Evaluating Proposed Research Projects

Before this new blood pressure medication could be administered to the residents of Sun Valley Care Center, the researchers would have been required to submit a proposal to the Institutional Review Board (IRB) at the university's medical school to conduct this study. The members of the IRB would review their research protocol to ensure proper protection for the human subjects to be used in the research project. In their review, the members of the IRB might use something like the following worksheet.

IRB WORKSHEET

. . . research will be founded on the four basic principles for human conduct: beneficence (doing good), nonmaleficence (not harming), respecting persons, and justice. The proposal is reviewed using six ethical norms for research involving human subjects founded on these principles. The criteria listed are conditions, each of which must be satisfied for a project to be ethically legitimate . . .

1. Good research design
   1.1 Based on a thorough knowledge of the scientific literature.
   1.2 Designed and based on results of experimentation at the pre-human level, if available.
   1.3 Conforms to generally accepted scientific principles.
   1.4 Expected to yield fruitful results for the good of society, unprocurable by other methods or means of study.
   1.5 Conducted so as to avoid all unnecessary physical and mental suffering and injury.
   1.6 Importance of the objective is in proportion to the inherent risk to the subject.
   1.7 Confidentiality: Every precaution is taken to respect the privacy of the subject and to minimize the impact of the study on the subject's physical and mental integrity and on the personality of the subject. In publication of the results, the doctor is obliged to preserve the accuracy of the results.
2. Balance of harm and benefit
   2.1 Degree of risk to be taken does not exceed that determined by the humanitarian importance of the problem to be solved by the experiment.
   2.2 Preceded by careful assessment of predictable risks in comparison with foreseeable benefits to the subject or to others.
   2.3 Concern for the interests of the subject always prevails over the interest of science and society.
3. Competence of the investigator(s)
   3.1 Investigator (or investigative team) has adequate training and skill to accomplish the purposes of the research.
   3.2 Supervision by a clinically competent medical person.
   3.3 A high degree of professionalism with evidence of responsibility for the human subject.

4. Informed consent
    4.1 Voluntary consent of the human subject is absolutely essential.
    4.2 Person involved has a legal capacity to give consent (OR if the person is legally incompetent, guardian consents; OR if a minor, responsible relative consent in addition to minor consent).
    4.3 Person or proxy acknowledges sufficient knowledge and comprehension of the elements of the research project (aims, methods, anticipated benefits, and potential hazards of the study and the discomfort it may entail).
    4.4 Free power of choice: The prospective subject or proxy is in no way highly dependent upon those who would be seeking consent.
    4.5 Person or proxy maintains the right to withdraw at any time without prejudice.
    4.6 Person or proxy will be informed that results of the study will be made available to him or her upon request.
    4.7 In instances of nontherapeutic experimentation, the proxy can give his consent only if the experiment entails no significant risk to the person's well-being. Moreover, the greater the person's incompetence and vulnerability, the greater the reasons must be to perform any medical experimentation, especially nontherapeutic.

5. Equitable selection of subjects
    5.1 Patient population: distribution of subjects is randomized and not solely those who are less advantaged.
    5.2 Protection of the vulnerable: no use of institutionalized subjects (prisoners) or persons with limited capacities to consent.
    5.3 Subjects should be volunteers.
    5.4 Subjects should be protected from arbitrary turn down without criteria.

6. Compensation for research-related injury
    6.1 Provision exists to discontinue research that is determined to likely result in injury, disability, or death to the experimental subject.
    6.2 Subjects who suffer physical, psychological, or social injury in the course of research shall be compensated 1) if the injury is primarily caused by such research and 2) if the injury exceeds that reasonably associated with such illness from which the subject may be suffering, as well as with treatment usually associated with such illness at the time the subject began participating in the research. (6).

From an ethical point of view, this IRB Worksheet is noteworthy in starting out with four fundamental ethical principles—beneficence, nonmaleficence, respecting persons, and justice. These principles are found in the Belmont Report, a landmark document on research ethics in the United States (5). The Belmont Report articulates respect for persons, beneficence (as including nonmaleficence), and justice as the basic ethical principles (5). Since, according to the Belmont Report, respect for persons requires that "individuals should be treated as autonomous agents" (5), these principles also mirror the ethical theory of principlism (see Chapter 1).

From these four fundamental ethical principles the IRB Worksheet derives six more specific norms for evaluating proposed research projects, namely, good research design, balance of harm and benefit, competence of the investigators, informed consent, equitable selection of subjects, and compensation for research-related injury. Exactly how do the six norms follow from the four fundamental principles?

The norms of good research design and competence of the investigator(s) are related to the principle of beneficence. For "without a competent investigator (or investigative team) and good research design, there will be no benefits forthcoming from the study" (7). These two norms are also related to the principle of nonmaleficence. This is so because "competent investigators and good research design also protect subjects from harm" (7).

The norm of balancing harm and benefit is derived from both the principle of beneficence (doing good) and the principle of nonmaleficence (not harming) (5).

The Belmont Report states that "respect for persons," that is autonomy, "requires that subjects, to the degree that they are capable, be given the opportunity to choose what shall or shall not happen to them, " an opportunity, which "is provided when adequate standards for informed consent are satisfied" (5).

The principle of justice requires fairness in the distribution of benefits and burdens. Justice is the foundation for the norm requiring an equitable selection of subjects. The "burdens" of research activity are the risks involved in experimentation, and it would be unfair to make the less advantaged and the vulnerable in society take all the risks. The principle of justice also serves as the foundation for the norm concerning compensation for research-related injury as compensation for undue burdens caused by participation in the research.

How does the blood pressure medication research project at Sun Valley Care Center stand up against these norms (and the more specific criteria for implementing them)? While we do not have enough detail about this research project to comment on each of the specific criteria listed in the IRB Worksheet, there are several points that stand out and deserve comment.

Any research project involves a balancing of benefits and risks for the human subjects participating in it (see IRB Worksheet 2.2). This is clearly illustrated in the case of Sun Valley Care Center. The occupational therapist Marilyn Stewart is cautioned by Sun Valley's administrator to watch for unusual symptoms or behavior in residents that may be caused by the medication being tested. These possible undesirable effects constitute the risks of this particular research study. These risks are counterbalanced by the expected benefits of the new medication, namely, that the residents will experience fewer of the side effects of the currently standard blood pressure medications.

There has been a problem with persons living in an institutional setting, such as a long-term care facility, being used as research subjects as a matter of convenience:

> Historically, nursing home patients were used as research participants disproportionately to their representation in the population, as were prisoners and other institutionalized groups, primarily for the convenience of the investigator. If the researcher can get all the subjects in one place, it is much easier to collect samples, do interviews, or conduct follow-up of the research. For example, it was much easier to get the consent of prisoners to participate by giving trivial amounts of money (or in some cases cartons of cigarettes) than it would have been to obtain consent from people in the community who have greater freedom. The studies were not particularly or especially relevant to problems of prisoners or problems of nursing home patients and therefore it was thought that this kind of selection bias was inequitable. (8)

Since medical research benefits society as a whole, there should, as a matter of justice, be an "equitable distribution of the burdens of participation in research" (8). This entails that "populations not be selected simply for the convenience of the investigator, but that they be selected for true representativeness related to the sample selection needs of the study" (8). Thus one criterion of legitimate research and experimentation is that subjects be selected equitably. No one group of persons should be used exclusively since this involves the possibility of exploiting certain groups in society, especially those who are less advantaged (see IRB Worksheet 5.1).

As far as we know, the new blood pressure medication is being tested *only* at Sun Valley Care Center. If, for example, Sun Valley were a county facility for indigent elderly persons (versus a nursing home where residents pay their own expenses), we would have good reason to worry that the research project was "using" poor people. However, we have no reason to think that Sun Valley is this type of facility. At the same time, we may worry that *only* the residents of Sun Valley are subjects in the research study. Are they being taken advantage of because they are in a nursing home? Why does the research study not include some elderly persons still living at home? (9).

Occupational therapist Marilyn Stewart notes a concern about the level of understanding the residents have of the project in which they are participating and the related issue of consent to participation. This is an issue that deserves extended examination.

Free and Informed Consent

A prominent principle in contemporary health care ethics is *patient autonomy*. Autonomy refers to self-determination. It affirms an individual's right to hold views, make choices, and take actions based on personal values and beliefs (see Chapter 1). The requirement to obtain the free and informed consent of an individual to participate in research and experimentation (see IRB Worksheet 4.1–4.4) is grounded in patient autonomy and concomitantly in the principle of respect for persons (5).

Federal regulations specify that the following information be provided to a potential research subject as basic elements of informed consent:

- A statement that the study involves research, an explanation of the purposes of the research and the expected duration of the subject's participation, a description of the procedures to be followed, and identification of any procedures that are experimental;
- A description of any reasonably foreseeable risks or discomforts to the subject;
- A description of any benefits to the subject or to others that may reasonably be expected from the research;
- A disclosure of appropriate alternative procedures or courses of treatment, if any, that might be advantageous to the subject;
- A statement describing the extent, if any, to which confidentiality of records identifying the subject will be maintained;
- For research involving more than minimal risk, an explanation as to whether any compensation and an explanation as to whether any medical treatments are available if injury occurs and, if so, what they consist of, or where further information may be obtained;
- An explanation of whom to contact for answers to pertinent questions about the research and research subjects' rights, and whom to contact in the event of a research-related injury to the subject; and

■ A statement that participation is voluntary, refusal to participate will involve no penalty or loss of benefits to which the subject is otherwise entitled, and the subject may discontinue participation at any time without penalty or loss of benefits to which the subject is otherwise entitled (10).

It is standard practice that a potential research subject (or his proxy) signs a written consent form to participate in the research project.

There are various challenges to obtaining truly free and informed consent from patients to participate in research projects. One challenge to "informed" consent is using language that is understandable to the potential research subjects in the consent forms that they must sign. Many consent forms "require the potential volunteer to 'synthesize information from complex or lengthy passages' . . . or to 'make high-level inferences or use specialized background knowledge' about medicine . . ." (11). Based on the results of the National Adult Literacy Survey (1993), it is estimated that only 3–20 percent of American adults have the reading skills needed to understand current research consent forms (11). Moreover, the survey indicated that people with a chronic illness, disability, or impairment have even lower levels of literacy skills than the total sample (11). This finding is especially relevant to the case involving the residents of Sun Valley Care Center in evaluating their ability to give informed consent to participation in the blood pressure medication research project.

As an illustration of the problem about using understandable language, consider the following excerpt from a consent form for trial of a new drug (IND):

> You will initially receive 50 milligrams (mg) of [IND] per kilogram (kg) of your body weight, followed by 25 mg/kg every 6 hours for 4 days, followed by 12.5 mg/kg every 6 hours for 6 days. (11)

This statement is not likely to give any clear information about dosage levels to someone who is not a health care worker. Consider a possible revision of it:

> The first dose will start right away. We will give bigger doses in the first 4 days, and smaller doses the last 6 days. Those are the same doses used for many years to treat other diseases. (11)

Not only is the language here much simpler and less technical, but the revision has the advantage of addressing a question potential research subjects will probably have. Few subjects are likely to want to know exactly how many milligrams of an experimental drug they will receive. They are more likely to want to know whether the dosage level is itself part of the experiment or if the same dose was found effective in previous research. The revision answers this question in a clear and straightforward way (11).

Other problems with obtaining truly informed consent concern the amount and detail of the information that is communicated. Studies indicate that the longer the consent form, the smaller the number of people that read the form in its entirety. This results in less, rather than more information being conveyed (11).

Further, extensive detail "usually enhances the subject's confusion" (12). Studies again indicate that the more elaborate the material presented to potential research subjects, the less they understand (12). Indeed, an investigator "conceivably could exploit his authority and knowledge and extract 'informed consent' by overwhelming the candidate-subject with information" (12). Researchers face the challenge of constructing consent forms that contain all the essential information but still are concise and relatively brief.

The communication process for obtaining a research subject's consent can be enhanced through the use of videotapes or portable flip cards that summarize key points in large print and contain graphics and diagrams (11). The latter might be especially helpful in working with the residents of Sun Valley Care Center, some of whom have poor eyesight and are hard of hearing. It has also been found that the procedure of "next day consent" improves the communication process. Soliciting consent takes place in a two-stage process, spread over at least 24 hours. This gives time for more information to be absorbed by potential research subjects and for discussion with their family members (11).

A potential subject's consent should be free as well as informed (see IRB Worksheet 4.1, 4.3). As pointed out by the U.S. Department of Health and Human Services, certain categories of potential research subjects "are likely to be vulnerable to coercion or undue influence, such as persons with acute or severe physical or mental illness, or persons who are economically or educationally disadvantaged" (13). The pressures that operate can be subtle ones. Consider, for example, the situation of patients in hospitals:

> Patients are psychologically predisposed to act in ways that please physicians. Not only do physicians possess a social role that makes them figures of authority, but an ill person feels very dependent on those who may possess the power to make him well. Thus, he will be inclined to go along with any suggestion or recommendation made by a physician. The ordinary patient, like the inmate in an institution, needs protection from the social and psychological pressures that are exerted by circumstances. Otherwise, the voluntariness of consent will be compromised. . . . (1)

Long-term care facilities (like Sun Valley Care Center in our case) and mental health facilities are *total institutions* within which "all aspects of a person's life are connected with the social structure" (1). In turn, there can be social forces operating to encourage and pressure a resident or patient to do what is expected of him or her (1). These subtle forms of pressure are undoubtedly the reason behind stipulation 4.3 in the IRB Worksheet: "The prospective subject or proxy is in no way highly dependent upon those who would be seeking consent."

Proxy Consent for Participation in Research and Experimentation

In our case, occupational therapist Marilyn Stewart notes that some of the residents of Sun Valley Care Center who are subjects in the blood pressure medication experiment are suffering from dementia, in varying degrees. Some of them may not have the capacity themselves to give free and informed consent to participate in the research project. Indeed, Marilyn raises the question of who made the decision about the residents participating in it.

In the case of mentally incapacitated adults and minors, proxy consent is recognized as legitimate. This is indicated in the IRB Worksheet: "Person involved has legal capacity to give consent (OR if person is legally incompetent, guardian consent; OR if a minor, responsible relative consent in addition to minor consent)" (2, 4). However, some ethicists draw a distinction between *consenting for oneself* and the role of *consenting for another*, placing restrictions on the latter type of consent.

Medical research and experimentation are considered therapeutic if it has the potential to benefit the subjects participating in the project. On the other hand, research and experimentation are classified as nontherapeutic if it is not expected to benefit the subjects themselves but will allow the researchers to gain knowledge that will benefit other patients. Some ethicists hold that proxy decision makers cannot licitly give consent to research and experimentation that is nontherapeutic in character (1, 14). Their reasoning is that a proxy decision maker has a duty to act in the best interests of the person he represents and for the welfare of that person (1, 14). Other ethicists take a less restrictive position, allowing for proxy consent to research and experimentation which poses only minimal risk to the subject (14). Point 4.7 of the IRB Worksheet given above allows for proxy consent for nontherapeutic research and experimentation, with certain qualifications: "In instances of nontherapeutic experimentation, the proxy can give his consent only if the experiment entails no significant risk to the person's well-being. Moreover, the greater the person's incompetence and vulnerability, the greater the reasons must be to perform any medical experimentation, especially nontherapeutic."

These stipulations and restrictions do not pose problems for the research project being carried on at Sun Valley Care Center. The new blood pressure medication being tested is expected to have fewer of the side effects many older persons experience with the current standard medications. If the new medication works as expected, it will clearly be of benefit to those taking it. Thus, this project qualifies as a therapeutic research for the residents participating in the project. Even those residents suffering from dementia may be included in the project, with the consent of the appropriate proxy decision maker.

CHAPTER SUMMARY

Key Terms and Concepts

principle of beneficence: the ethical duty to act in ways that help people and promote their welfare.

principle of nonmaleficence: the ethical duty to act in ways that do not cause harm to people.

principle of respect for persons: a principle requiring that persons be treated as autonomous agents.

principle of autonomy: self-determination; an individual's right to hold views, make choices, and take actions based on personal values and beliefs.

principle of justice: a principle concerning fairness in the distribution of benefits, burdens, and resources.

therapeutic research and experimentation: research and experimentation that has the potential to benefit the subjects participating in it.

nontherapeutic research and experimentation: research and experimentation that is not expected to benefit the subjects participating in it, but will allow researchers to gain knowledge to benefit other patients.

Key Points

- Abuses have occurred in the past with the use of human beings in medical research and experimentation. These abuses have resulted in the formulation of codes of research ethics and the establishment of IRBs (institutional review boards).

- An IRB will review proposed research projects using such norms as good research design, the balance of harm and benefit involved in the project, the competence of the investigator(s), informed consent, whether the subjects of the experiment have been selected equitably, and provision for compensation for research-related injury. These norms follow from the ethical principles of beneficence, nonmaleficence, respect for persons and autonomy, and justice. More specific criteria are developed for implementing these general norms.

- The process of obtaining informed consent from a potential research subject involves giving the individual a description of the expected benefits of a research project and its potential discomforts and risks, of alternatives that might be advantageous, and of the procedures to be followed. Subjects must also be informed that they may refuse to participate in the project. Normally all of this information is provided in a written consent form.

- Challenges in obtaining informed consent include presenting information in language that is understandable to potential research subjects, and constructing consent forms that contain all essential information while still being concise and relatively brief.

- Consent to participate in research projects should be free as well as informed. Researchers need to be sensitive to subtle coercive forces that can influence the consent of patients and residents. These coercive forces include the state of dependency of patients and residents on their health care providers and the fact that all aspects of a resident's life in, for example, a long-term care facility are connected with the institution's social structure.

- Proxy consent for participation in medical research and experimentation is considered legitimate in the case of minors and mentally incapacitated adults. However, ethicists tend to limit the range of legitimate proxy consent to projects that involve only minimal risk for the participating subject, or sometimes more narrowly to projects that are therapeutic in nature.

FOR FURTHER DISCUSSION

1. Rose Stillman and Michael Bauer are occupational therapists who work at a university medical center. They have both become interested in music therapy. They want to conduct a research project that will consist in playing Gregorian chant to agitated Alzheimer's patients and observing them to determine if the music has a calming effect on their behavior (15).

    Divide the class into two groups. Let the first group represent the researchers Rose Stillman and Michael Bauer, and let the second group represent an Institutional Review Board (IRB) for the facility at which their research project will be conducted.

The researchers should construct a proposal for their project to submit for IRB approval.

This group will need to develop the details of the projected research project beyond the description given. (HINT: The proposal should include the following information: the purpose of the research project and the researcher's hypothesis; methods and procedures for conducting the research; the number, age range, and gender of participants, and how and where they will be recruited/selected; potential benefits and risks of the project; how the data collected will be handled in terms of confidentiality; the credentials of the researchers; an informed consent form.)

The second group should role play a meeting of the IRB to discuss and approve or reject the proposal submitted to them. Does the proposal address and satisfy the various criteria for legitimate experimentation on humans set out in this chapter?

2. When the disease AIDS became prominent, complaints were voiced about the slowness of the U.S. Food and Drug Administration (FDA) in testing and approving drugs which might benefit persons with AIDS. Should patients with life-limiting illnesses have access to any drug they might wish to try, even if research and testing on it have not yet been completed? Should we be guided in these decisions primarily by the ethical principle of autonomy or the ethical principle of nonmaleficence? (16).

3. It is possible to sustain by technological means the vital functions of an individual who has suffered brain death. It has been proposed that such legally dead human beings be sustained specifically for use as subjects in medical research experiments (17–19). From an ethical point of view, do you see any problems with doing this?

References

1. Ronald Munson, "Medical Experimentation and Informed Consent" in *Intervention and Reflection: Basic Issues in Medical Ethics*, 5th ed., ed. Ronald Munson (Belmont, CA: Wadsworth, 1996).

2. Alexander M. Capron, "Human Experimentation" in *Medical Ethics*, ed. Robert M. Veatch (Boston, MA: Jones & Bartlett, 1989).

3. *Trials of War Criminals Before the Nuremberg Military Tribunals Under Control Council Law No. 10*, vol. 2 (Washington, DC: United States Government Printing Office, 1949).

4. Adopted by the 18th World Medical Assembly, Helsinki, Finland, 1964; revised 1975, 1983, 1989. Reprinted in the *Encyclopedia of Bioethics*, rev. ed. (New York, NY: Macmillan, 1995).

5. National Commission for the Protection of Human Subjects of Biomedical and Behavioral Research, "*The Belmont Report Ethical Principles and Guidelines for the Protection of Human Subjects of Research* (1979)." http://www.hhs.gov/ohrp/humansubjects/guidance/belmont.html. Accessed April 2016.

6. *Research Manual,* Mercy Medical Center, Dubuque, IA (1996).

7. Robert J. Levine and Karen Lebacqz, "Ethical Considerations in Clinical Trials," *Clinical Pharmacology and Therapeutics* 25/5-2 (May 1979): 728–741.

8. Christine Cassel, "Ethical Issues in the Conduct of Research in Long Term Care," *The Gerontologist* 28 Suppl. (1988): 90–96.

9. Christine Cassel, "Research in Nursing Homes Ethical Issues," *Journal of the American Geriatrics Society* 33/11 (November 1985): 795–99.

10. *"Code of Federal Regulations, Title 45 Public Welfare; Department of Health and Human Services, Part 46 Protection of Human Subjects, 46.116 General Requirements for Informed Consent."* http://www.hhs.gov/ohrp/humansubjects/guidance/45cfr46.html. Accessed April 2016.

11. William L. Freeman, "Making Research Consent Forms Informative and Understandable: The Experience of the Indian Health Service," *Cambridge Quarterly of Health care Ethics* 3 (1994): 510–21.

12. Franz J. Ingelfinger, "Informed (But Uneducated) Consent," *New England Journal of Medicine* 287/9 (August 31, 1972): 465–66.

13. United States Department of Health and Human Services, *Policy for the Protection of Human Research Subjects* 46.111 (7b) in 46 FR 8386, January 26, 1981, 48 FR 9269, March 4, 1983.

14. Benedict M. Ashley, OP and Kevin D. O'Rourke, OP, *Healthcare Ethics: A Theological Analysis*, 3rd ed. (St. Louis, MO: Catholic Health Association, 1989).

15. Dr. Alice Cash, "*Healing Music Enterprises.*" http://www.healingmusicenterprises.com. Accessed April 2016.

16. "Drug Testing, Autonomy, and Access to Unapproved Drugs" in *Intervention and Reflection: Basic Issues in Medical Ethics*, 5th ed. ed. Ronald Munson (Belmont, CA: Wadsworth, 1996).

17. Willard Gaylin, "Harvesting the Dead," *Harpers* 249 (September 1974): 23–26.

18. Ronald A. Carson, Jaime L. Frias, and Richard J. Melker, "Case Study: Research With Brain-Dead Children," *IRB* 3/1 (1981): 5–6.

19. Susan R. Martyn, "Using the Brain Dead for Medical Research," *Utah Law Review* (1986): 1–28.

Chapter 18

Stem Cell Research

Some issues in health care ethics, such as confidentiality or forgoing life-sustaining treatments, are perennial ones. Other issues emerge with the advent of new diseases (such as acquired immunodeficiency syndrome [AIDS]) or with new developments in scientific and medical research (such as the Human Genome Project). One issue that has become prominent in the 21st century is stem cell research.

In this chapter you will learn:

- Basic biological information about stem cells;
- Ethical questions about deriving stem cells from early embryos;
- Ethical concerns surrounding cloning human beings to obtain stem cells.

Case Study

Tim Murphy, 78, was widowed 5 years ago. Since the death of his wife, he has been using home health care services. His mobility is limited because of arthritis and, as he puts it, a "worn out" hip and knee. Within the last year, the home health care staff visiting him has noticed that he has slowed down considerably. Lately, he coughs when he drinks liquids, which makes the staff suspect swallowing problems.

The staff of the home health care service persuades Tim to make an appointment with a neurologist, who diagnoses Tim as in early stage Parkinson's disease. Arrangements are made for Tim to work with a speech therapist about his swallowing problem.

Tim's daughter, Martha, accompanies him to see the speech therapist, Rebecca Smith. Rebecca discusses with Tim and Martha how his diet can be managed to assist him in swallowing. Rebecca also mentions a research project going on at a local university medical center for patients with Parkinson's disease. The research project involves a therapy using stem cells, replacing the dopamine-producing cells in the brains of Parkinson's patients. Rebecca offers to contact the medical center to see if Tim can be enrolled in the project.

Initially, Martha is excited about the availability of a therapy that could help her father and prevent the progress of his Parkinson's disease. Martha has a close friend whose mother suffered from Parkinson's disease for 10 years before her death, and she knows how devastating a disease it can be.

At the same time, Martha remembers from her college biology course the controversy that has surrounded the development of therapies from stem cells. Martha has always considered herself to be "pro-life," and she wonders about the ethics of using therapies dependent on stem cells. For this reason, she tells Rebecca Smith that she wants to learn more about these therapies and to consult with her pastor before pursuing the experimental treatment for her father.

The Science of Stem Cells: The Basics

The various tissues and organs of the human body consist of specialized cells adapted to perform certain functions; for example, blood cells, heart cells, muscle cells, and brain cells. Stem cells are cells that are capable of dividing and renewing themselves for long periods, are unspecialized, and can give rise to specialized cell types (1).

There are various sources of stem cells. They can be obtained from embryos, adult tissues, umbilical cord blood, and amniotic fluid (with the stem cells lodging in the placenta) (2, 3). They have also been found in women's menstrual blood (4); indeed, services exist for women to bank the stem cells in their menstrual blood for future use (5, 6). It is likewise possible to genetically reprogram adult cells to an embryonic stem cell-like state. These are called induced pluripotent stem cells. (1) Although stem cells can be obtained from fetuses (2), this is not currently an area of emphasis in stem cell research. It is the use of embryonic stem cells that has become a topic of intense ethical debate.

Embryonic stem cells are derived from embryos that have developed from eggs fertilized in vitro. Often the embryos were created for reproductive purposes and subsequently donated for research. At the blastocyst stage of development, which occurs around day 4 or 5, the blastocyst has three structures: the trophoblast, an outer ring of cells that will develop into the placenta; the blastocoel, a hollow cavity inside the blastocyst; and the inner cell mass, that will develop into the fetus. Human embryonic stem cells are isolated by transferring the inner cell mass into a laboratory culture dish. Obviously, this destroys the embryo as such. Ultimately, the intent is to coax the stem cells into differentiating into the desired tissue, which would then be placed into the body of the recipient (1, 7).

However, such a transplantation faces the well-known problem of immune rejection because the stem cells derived from the embryos will be genetically different from the recipient's genome. One method for overcoming this problem, which researchers are exploring, is cloning. In a procedure known as somatic cell nuclear transfer (SCNT), the nuclear DNA is removed from an unfertilized ovum and replaced with the nuclear DNA of a somatic cell (a nonreproductive body cell) from the intended recipient of the procedure. The new cell receives a jolt of electricity to begin cell division and growth. When the appropriate stage of embryonic development is reached, the aforementioned procedure for obtaining stem cells will be used. This procedure is known as "therapeutic cloning" to distinguish it from "reproductive cloning," the potential use of cloning to produce a live born child (2, 8). However, SCNT will not give a perfect genetic match "because mitochondrial genes would come from the donor egg cell," and thus "there is a potential for exposure of foreign mitochondrial proteins that could cause tissue rejection" (2). Hence, "patients may still require taking antirejection medications though the dosage may be lower" (2).

First and foremost, there is intense interest in stem cell research because of therapies that could be developed. Stem cells could generate cells and tissues to treat a variety of diseases, such as Parkinson's, Alzheimer's, spinal cord injury, stroke, burns, heart disease, diabetes, and arthritis (1). Further, the need for transplantable tissues and organs exceeds the available supply, and tissues and organs grown from stem cells might help meet this need (1). Studies of human embryonic stem cells are expected to yield information about the events that occur during human development, especially cell differentiation to form tissues and organs. This, in turn, could provide insight into serious medical conditions such as cancer and birth defects, which are due to abnormal cell division and differentiation (1). Finally, stem cells could be used to produce differentiated cells for testing new drugs (1).

Stem cell research is a rapidly developing area of scientific research. For this reason, supplementary resources should be consulted to become informed about the latest work and advances in stem cell research.

The Ethics of Stem Cell Research

Stem cell research is often presented in a black and white fashion: one is either for it or against it. From an ethical point of view, distinctions must be made among different types of stem cell research.

Research utilizing stem cells derived from sources other than embryos (or aborted fetuses)—stem cells obtained from adult tissues, umbilical cord blood, amniotic fluid and the placenta, and women's menstrual blood—has not been controversial ethically (8–10), although such research must be conducted in accord with accepted standards for medical research and experimentation on humans (see Chapter 17). When induced pluripotent stem cells (iPs cells) were first developed, researchers created lentiviruses which contained the reprogramming genes. The creation of these viruses required the use of hek293 helper cells, which were embryonic in origin. This was ethically controversial. However, researchers have moved away from this methodology and iPs cells can now be created without the use of viruses or helper cells (11). Thus, in terms of the current practice of stem cell research, it is embryonic stem cell research and therapeutic cloning that are ethically controversial.

Obtaining stem cells from embryos involves the destruction of early stage embryos. Thus one's judgment about the ethical permissibility of embryonic stem cell research is dependent on one's views on the human and moral status of the early stage embryo (see the discussion of this issue in Chapter 3). In this regard, three basic positions have emerged in the literature on embryonic stem cell research (12).

One position is that the early stage embryo from which stem cells are obtained is simply organic material and has no moral status at all (12). Specifically, it is argued that "the blastocysts before implantation cannot be harmed by being destroyed" because "to be harmed means to have an interest or interests defeated" (12). But " For a being to have an interest, this being must have beliefs, desires, expectations, aims, and purposes" and "the nervous system of such early embryos is not developed enough for this" (12). Consequently, "because they are not the subjects of interests, such early embryos cannot be the subjects of basic rights that protect interests" (12). In sum, this position sees no ethical problems with destroying embryos to obtain stem cells.

A second position is represented by the Ethics Advisory Board of the bio-technology corporation Geron. On the issue of the human and moral status of the embryo and fetus, it adopted a developmental view. This view, while acknowledging that human life begins at conception, holds that human person-hood and full moral status is a later development. (13). In other words, "moral status is understood developmentally: as the conceptus develops from blastocyst to fetus and beyond so too does moral status grow" (13). The Ethics Advisory Board affirmed that "a fundamental principle of respect for human life applies at all states of human development" (13) but proposed that "early embryonic tissue is respected by ensuring that it is used with care only in research that incorporates substantive values such as reduction of human suffering" (13). The Board judged that the purposes of human embryonic stem cell research, in terms of "its potential to contribute to fundamental knowledge of human devel-opment and to medical and pharmaceutical interventions to alleviate suffering" do "provide such substantive values" (13).

A third position is that, from the time of conception/fertilization, the embryo is a human being with full moral status, and concomitantly, has interests and rights that must be respected (9, 12, 14). On this view, harvesting embryonic stem cells "involves the deliberate killing of innocent human beings, a gravely immoral act" (9).

Apart from the issue of the status of the early stage embryo, a utilitarian line of argument (see Chapter 1) has been offered to support embryonic stem cell research:

> . . . proponents contend that the end result of sacrificing embryos
> to harvest their stem cells would be so overwhelmingly positive for a

large number of suffering people that it must be the right thing to do. The moral calculus points to the alleged potential good of treating or healing illnesses such as Parkinson's disease, Alzheimer's disease, or diabetes. According to a commonly-heard argument, without the use of embryonic stem cells critical research cannot move forward, and the amelioration of human suffering and the saving of lives will be thwarted. The end goal of healing justifies the destruction of human embryos to procure stem cells. Healing is regarded as the "greatest good" which will usher in the most happiness or pleasure for the greatest number of people. Therefore, it should be pursued at the expense of embryonic life. (15)

In reply, it might be pointed out that proponents of this line of argument tend to downplay the therapeutic potential of non-embryonic stem cells (15). Such stem cells are already being used to provide therapies for human patients with a wide range of health problems:

- Cancers (e.g., brain cancer, ovarian cancer, breast cancer, skin cancer, leukemia, lymphoma);
- Autoimmune diseases (e.g., juvenile diabetes, lupus, scleroderma, Crohn's disease, multiple sclerosis);
- Cardiovascular disease (e.g., acute heart damage, chronic coronary artery disease);
- Ocular disease (e.g., corneal regeneration);
- Immunodeficiencies (e.g., severe combined immunodeficiency syndrome);
- Neural degenerative diseases and syndromes (e.g., Parkinson's disease, spinal cord injury, stroke damage);
- Anemias and other blood conditions (e.g., sickle cell anemia, thalassemia);
- Wounds and injuries (e.g., limb gangrene, jawbone replacement);
- Metabolic disorders (e.g., Hurler's syndrome);
- Liver disease (e.g., liver cirrhosis, chronic liver failure) and end-stage bladder disease (16).

Thus, it is argued that the therapeutic good of stem cell research can be achieved without destroying human embryos.

A second utilitarian line of argument focuses on the use of spare frozen embryos from fertility clinics (17). It is applicable even if one considers the early stage embryo to be a human being.

The process of in vitro fertilization (IVF) typically involves retrieving and fertilizing a number of ova. However, not all the embryos created are transferred to a woman's body at a given time to try to achieve a pregnancy; this is done to prevent multifetal pregnancies. Remaining embryos may be frozen for later use. However, frozen embryos may become "spare" if a couple achieves the child they want and does not want to keep any remaining frozen embryos for future attempts at having children. Or sometimes the IVF procedure simply does not work to achieve a pregnancy and a discouraged couple gives up trying, although some frozen embryos they have created remain. Such spare frozen embryos are sometimes donated to infertile couples for adoption or they may simply be destroyed (see Chapter 4). Thus the argument is made that, if spare frozen embryos are destined to be destroyed anyway, they ought to be donated for stem cell research that will benefit other people (9, 17).

One ethicist has set out essentially the same kind of argument by using a maxim he denominates the "nothing-is-lost" principle and extending it from certain kinds of conflict cases to the case of spare frozen embryos destined to be destroyed (18):

> The nothing-is-lost principle, as understood by Outka, is intended to permit the use of lethal force in cases of conflict. In Outka's formulation, "One may directly kill when two conditions obtain: (a) the innocent will die in any case; and (b) other innocent life will be saved." In the case of embryos, Outka wishes to extend the principle in the following way: One may directly kill if "(a) nothing more is lost, and (b) less is lost, or at least someone is saved."
>
> Thus, in the case of embryos left over from IVF, research upon which might be useful to saving lives, Outka writes, "They will die, unimplanted in any case. (Nothing more will be lost by their becoming subjects of research.) Thus Outka's conclusion, that, since some lives might be saved, and nothing will be lost, it is permissible to experiment on embryos already alive, but without any hope of being brought to maturation. (18)

In reply, those who are unqualifiedly opposed to embryonic stem cell research point out that "our society does not permit lethal experiments on terminally ill patients or condemned prisoners on the pretext that they will soon die anyway" (9) Similarly, "the fact that an embryonic human being is at risk of being abandoned by his or her parents gives no individual or government a right to directly kill that human being first" (9).

Ethical Issues in Cloning for Stem Cell Research

Cloning for stem cell research ("therapeutic cloning") uses the process of somatic cell nuclear transfer (SCNT). No sperm is involved in SCNT. This has raised the question of whether a new human embryo, properly speaking, is produced through this process.

> Other opponents of SCNT express concern that it creates human life only to destroy it for research purposes. In fact, no new life is created by SCNT. It works entirely with the ordinary body cells of an already-living person. It no more creates human life than does growing someone's skin cells in tissue culture . . .
>
> SCNT does not entail fertilization of an egg with a sperm. It does not involve conception of a new human life. Instead, it awakens the developmental potential in the genome of cells from a person conceived years ago. (19)

If no new human life is created through SCNT, then the ethical objection that SCNT "creates human life only to destroy it for research purposes" does not hold up.

However, issue is taken with this claim on biological grounds. Critics contend that cloning through SCNT "produces the same result" as fertilization "by combining what is normally combined and activated in fertilization, that is, the full genetic code plus the ovular cytoplasm" (18). That a human embryo is indeed created through SCNT has been affirmed by a prominent embryonic stem cell researcher, James Thomson:

> If you create an embryo by nuclear transfer, and you give it to somebody who didn't know where it came from, there would be no test you could do on that embryo to say where it came from. It is what it is . . . . But by any reasonable definition, at least at some frequency, you're creating an embryo. If you try to define it away, you're being disingenuous. (20)

Further, it is pointed out that SCNT was used to create Dolly the cloned sheep (2), and Dolly was clearly a "new organism." The same procedure of SCNT is used to create an embryo whether it will be used for reproductive purposes or to obtain stem cells. The only difference in the two cases is what is done with the embryo once it is created.

A reservation about cloning for stem cell research is its potential exploitative impact on women (21). Thousands, possibly millions of ova will be required for

SCNT research (21), and these must be donated by women. Multiple ova, not just one, will be extracted from a woman at a given time. The "extraction of multiple eggs involves both ovarian suppression and what is known as 'ovarian hyperstimulation' using powerful hormones into a woman's body to manipulate it into producing many—often a dozen or more—eggs at a time rather than the normal one or two" (21). However, this procedure can result in ovarian hyperstimulation syndrome (OHSS). In its mild form, OHSS causes symptoms of abdominal discomfort, ovarian enlargement, nausea, and vomiting. In its more severe forms, OHSS can result in loss of fertility, kidney, or multiple organ failure, and even death (21). Ethically, procedures that pose serious risks of harm to persons violate the principle of nonmaleficence (see Chapter 1). Further, there is concern that SCNT may cause the emergence of a "market in eggs" (21), and that poorer women in need of money may be attracted to egg donation for stem cell research (22).

Indeed, an international organization has been established called Hands Off Our Ovaries with the mission to "seek a moratorium on egg extraction for research purposes until such time as global discourse and scientific research yields information sufficient to establish adequate informed consent" (23). Such informed consent should include "assessments regarding the short and long term medical risk of egg harvesting," with FDA investigation of "the 25 deaths and over 6,000 complaints of medical complications associated with the drug, Lupron" (23). In addition, informed consent requires studies of the long- and short-term risks of Ovarian Hyper-Stimulation Syndrome (OHSS) (23), and long-term studies of "possible connections between egg extraction procedures and uterine, ovarian and other reproductive cancers, infertility, adverse birth outcomes, and other iatrogenic conditions" (23).

CHAPTER SUMMARY

Key Terms and Concepts

stem cell: cells that are capable of dividing and renewing themselves for long periods, are unspecialized, and can give rise to specialized cell types.

somatic cell nuclear transfer (SCNT): a procedure in which the nuclear DNA is removed from an unfertilized ovum and replaced with that of a somatic cell (a non-reproductive body cell) from a donor.

therapeutic cloning: the use of somatic cell nuclear transfer (SCNT) to produce embryonic stem cells that will be a closer match genetically for the intended recipient of the stem cell therapy.

Key Points

- First and foremost, there is intense interest in stem cell research because of therapies that could be developed for a variety of diseases. Organs and tissues grown from stem cells might help meet transplantation needs. Embryonic stem cell research could also yield.information about human development and insight into serious medical conditions due to abnormal cell division and differentiation. Stem cells could likewise be used to produce differentiated cells for testing new drugs.

- There are various sources of stem cells: embryos, fetuses, adult tissues, umbilical cord blood, amniotic fluid (with the stems cell lodging in the placenta), and menstrual blood. It is likewise possible to genetically reprogram adult cells to an embryonic stem cell-like state (induced pluripotent stem cells).

- Tissues and organs created from embryonic stem cells will face the problem of immune rejection because they will be genetically different from the recipient. One method that researchers are exploring for overcoming this problem is cloning, using the technique of SCNT. However, SCNT does not produce an exact genetic match so that some degree of immune rejection will remain.

- One's judgment about the ethical permissibility of embryonic stem cell research depends on one's views on the human and moral status of the early stage embryo.

- An argument in favor of embryonic stem cell research has been offered on utilitarian grounds. Opponents of embryonic stem cell research maintain that the therapeutic good of stem cell research can be achieved using non-embryonic stem cells.

- Even if one considers the early stage embryo to be a human being, some argue that it is still permissible to use spare frozen embryos from fertility clinics in stem cell research because they will be destroyed anyway. Those who are unqualifiedly opposed to embryonic stem cell research point out that our society does not permit lethal experiments on terminally ill patients or condemned prisoners on the grounds that they will soon die anyway.

- Some claim that using somatic cell nuclear transfer (SCNT) to produce stem cells does not involve the creation of a new human embryo properly speaking. However, this claim has been challenged on biological grounds.

- Reservations about cloning for stem cell research include its potentially exploitative impact on women who have to donate the ova to be used in the procedure.

FOR FURTHER DISCUSSION

1. Despite some opposition, embryonic stem cell research is going forward. Going back to the chapter's opening case study, suppose that Martha learns that the proposed therapy for her father was developed using embryonic stem cells and that she personally considers embryonic stem cell research to be ethically impermissible. Given that Martha had no part in how the therapy was developed and given its potential for significant benefit for her father, do you think it is ethically permissible for Martha to agree to the use of this therapy even though she regards the way it was developed as ethically wrong?

2. "Some opponents of SCNT contend that it is not pro-life. Former U.S. Senator Jack Danforth, an ordained Episcopal priest with unassailable prolife credentials, provided the best answer to this concern when he said, '*The proposal to criminalize cell regeneration research calls for a choice between two understandings of human life. On one hand, we have the millions of people who suffer from ALS, Alzheimer's, juvenile diabetes, Parkinson's, spinal cord injuries and cancer—and the loved ones who care for them and suffer by their sides. On the other hand, we have tiny bundles of unfertilized cells existing in Petri dishes. Supporters of the legislation should explain to the afflicted and their loved ones why they care more about those cell bundles than they do about the people*'" (19). Do you find this a plausible line of argument? What might opponents of embryonic stem cell research and therapeutic cloning say in response?

3. Research current therapeutic successes using embryonic and nonembryonic stem cells. Does this information change your views on embryonic stem cell research? On how we should allocate funding for stem cell research?

References

1. National Institutes of Health, *Stem Cell Information: Stem Cell Basics.* http://stemcells.nih.gov/info/basics/pages/basics1.aspx. Accessed March 2016.

2. John Paul II Medical Research Institute, *Stem Cell Education.* http://www.jp2mri.org. Accessed March 2016.

3. Nikhil Swaminathan, "New Source of Stem Cells: Amniotic Fluid," *Scientific American* (January 7, 2007). http://www.scientificamerican.com/article/new-source-of-stem-cells. Accessed March 2016

4. Alison Motluk, "*Menstrual Blood Could Be Rich Source of Stem Cells.*" http://www.newscientist.com/article/dn12924-menstrual-blood-cold-be-rich-source-of-stem-cells. Accessed March 2016.

5. CryoCell International, *Banking Menstrual Stem Cells.* http://www.cryocell .com/menstrual/stem-cells. Accessed March 2016.

6. Express Healthcare, *LifeCell Brings Menstrual Blood Stem Cell Banking to India.* http://archivehealthcare.financialexpress.com/201104/market13.shtml. Accessed March 2016.

7. News@UW-Madison, *Wisconsin Scientists Culture Elusive Embryonic Stem Cells,* November 5, 1998. http://www.news.wisc.edu/wisconsin-scientists-culture-elusive-embryonic-stem-cells. Accessed March 2016.

8. NeuroTalk, *Biology 101: An Explanation of Stem Cells and Cloning.* http:// neurotalk.psychcentral.com/showthread.php?t=3759. Accessed March 2016.

9. United States Conference of Catholic Bishops, *On Embryonic Stem Cell Research,* 2008. http://www.usccb.org/issues-and-action/human-life-and-dignity/stem-cell-research. Accessed March 2016.

10. United States Conference of Catholic Bishops, *Ethical and Religious Directives for Catholic Health Care Services,* 5th ed. (2009), no. 66. http://www.usccb. org. Accessed March 2016.

11. E-mail correspondence with Anant Kamath, Cellular Engineering Technologies, Coralville, IA. March 28, 2016.

12. EuroStemCell, *Human Embryonic Stem Cell Research and Ethics* (March 4, 2011). http://www.eurostemcell.org. Accessed March 2016.

13. Geron Ethics Advisory Board, "Research With Human Embryonic Stem Cells: Ethical Considerations," in *The Stem Cell Controversy Debating the Issues,* eds. Michael Ruse and Christopher A. Pynes (Amherst, NY: Prometheus Books, 2003), 107–19.

14. Bernard Lo and Lindsay Parham, "Ethical Issues in Stem Cell Research," *Endocrine Review* 30/3 (May 2009): 204–13.

15. Dennis P. Hollinger, *Stem Cells & Our Moral Culture.* https://cbhd.org/ print/content/stem-cells-our-moral-culture. Accessed March 2016.

16. Stem Cell Research Facts.org, *Benefits of Adult Stem Cells for Human Patients.* http://www.stemcellresearchfacts.org/treatment-list. Accessed March 2016.

17. Dennis M. Sullivan and Aaron Costerisan, "Complicity and Stem Cell Research: Countering the Utilitarian Argument," *Ethics & Medicine* 24/3 (2008): 151–58.

18. Robert P. George and Christopher Tollefsen, *Embryo a Defense of Human Life* (New York, NY: Doubleday, 2008).

19. William B. Neaves, "Stem Cells From Somatic Cell Nuclear Transfer: Research to Unlock the Body's Potential for Self-Repair," *Missouri Medicine* 102/1 (January/February 2005): 14–17.

20. Alan Boyle, *Stem Cell Pioneer Does a Reality Check: James Thomson on Science and Morality.* http://www.nbcnews.com/id/8303756.ns/health-cloning_and_stem_cells/t/stem-cell-pioneer-does-reality-check/#.VvKz43pY7XE. Accessed March 2016.

21. Diane Beeson, *Testimony to the House Government Reform Subcommittee on Criminal Justice, Drug Policy and Human Resources—Hearing on Stem Cell Research* (March 7, 2006). http://www.handsoffourovaries.com>Commentary. Accessed March 2016.

22. Core European Seminar, *Human Egg Trading and the Exploitation of Women* (Brussels, June 30, 2005). http://www.handsoffourovaries.com>Commentary. Accessed March 2016.

23. Hands Off Our Ovaries, *Mission.* http://handsoffourovaries.com/mission.htm. Accessed March 2016.

Index